Helping the Youthful Offender: Individual and Group Therapies That Work

THE CHILD & YOUTH SERVICES SERIES

EDITOR-IN-CHIEF

JEROME BEKER, *Director and Professor, Center for Youth Development and Research, University of Minnesota*

Helping
the Youthful Offender:
Individual and Group
Therapies That Work

William B. Lewis

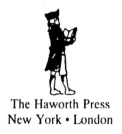

The Haworth Press
New York • London

Helping the Youthful Offender: Individual and Group Therapies That Work has also been published as *Child & Youth Services*, Volume 11, Number 2 1989.

The Haworth Press, Inc., 10 Alice Street, Binghamton, NY 13904-1580
EUROSPAN/Haworth, 3 Henrietta Street, London WC2E 8LU England

Library of Congress Cataloging-in-Publication Data

Lewis, William B.
   Helping the youthful offender : individual and group therapies that work/William B. Lewis.
   p. cm.
   "Has also been published as Child & youth services, Volume 11, Number 2, 1989" – T.p. verso.
   Includes bibliographical references.
   ISBN: 1-56024-127-6 (pbk.)
   1. Rehabilitation of juvenile delinquents – California. 2. Social work with delinquents and criminals – California. I. Title.
HV9105.C2L49   1989
364.3'6'09794 – dc20   89-33070
                                                                                          CIP

DEDICATED TO:

Gerald Spencer, the Superintendent whose encouragement nurtured my work and whose vision enabled California Youth Authority institutions to create effective treatment environments.

Helping the Youthful Offender: Individual and Group Therapies That Work

CONTENTS

ABOUT THE AUTHOR

William B. Lewis, PhD, is currently Consulting Psychologist for San Mar Group Homes in Bloomington, Ontario, and Montclair, California, and for Mental Health Systems, Inc. in San Diego, California. Since completing an internship in clinical psychology in 1952, his career has included clinical practice, teaching, writing, treatment program development, and correctional administration. He began a long and distinguished career with the Department of the Youth Authority in California as a senior psychologist and retired as Assistant Chief of Institutions and Camps in 1983. Dr. Lewis developed the California Youth Authority's first specialized treatment program for emotionally disturbed delinquent youth. He also developed the Department's first programs of milieu therapy, small group counseling, staff relationship groups, community counseling, and the case conference approach to classification. His innovations in correctional treatment can be observed today in institutions, camps, and parole offices not only throughout the California Youth Authority, but across the nation as well.

Foreword

The California Youth Authority in 1988 is one of the nation's most sophisticated correctional agencies. Its many institutions, forestry camps, and parole offices offer a variety of specialized treatment approaches for youthful offenders with different needs.

Thirty-two years ago, in 1956, such programs did not exist. That was the year that Bill Lewis finished his duty tour with the United States Navy Medical Service Corps and accepted a position as clinical psychologist at the Youth Authority's Paso Robles School. Two years later he received the Department's Outstanding Employee Award for having designed and implemented its first specialized treatment program for emotionally disturbed youthful offenders.

Bill discovered early that the treatment skills of one clinician do not reach very far in a population of several hundred. He also found that traditional approaches to therapy often did not work with delinquent youth and, in fact, sometimes made them worse. Consequently, he shifted his emphasis to program development, staff training, and evolving individual and group therapies that *would* work.

Until his retirement as assistant chief of institutions and camps in 1983, Bill continued to create new programs to meet the needs of youths with special problems. Among these were a five-program special treatment complex (Unit II) at Youth Training School in Ontario, California and the drug-alcohol treatment program at the Fred C. Nelles School in Whittier. His ideas have been expanded in many specialized treatment programs throughout the Department today.

Dr. Lewis was a pioneer in assisting the California Youth Authority in carrying out its mission to protect society through the detention and rehabilitation of youthful offenders. His methods, as described in this book, may prove equally useful to others in the "people work" business.

C. A. Terhune, Director
Department of the Youth Authority
State of California

Preface

Dear Reader:

I found myself reliving some exciting personal memories as I read Dr. Lewis's book and his lively vignettes of the troubled and delinquent kids he treated at Paso Robles. You see, I was there when those stories unfolded. I knew all of the kids he describes and followed their progress at the time. Bill would bend my ear about each of them as he taught me the same concepts he presents here for all of you.

Although I had already spent a number of years as a correctional worker when these stories took place, my concept of what I wanted to do with my youthful clients was ambiguous (a state of affairs I still find typical among young people working the correctional field). I had no "method" to use in order to communicate with my charges effectively and consistently. Using the concepts Bill so clearly outlines in the pages of this book, I learned how to make a connection with those "bad boys" that has never ceased enriching my life.

In some ways, Bill's book is old-fashioned. In recent years, treatment programs in youth-correctional facilities have been losing out in the battle over budget priorities. They have given way to the building of higher walls, the purchasing of heavier weaponry for the guards, and the use of more "time" (incarceration for the sake of incarceration). To advocates of these "modern" trends, Bill's ideas on "treatment" and "counseling" are likely to fall on deaf ears. People (such as me) who align themselves with Bill are supposedly naive, and "soft on crime." The field of corrections seems much more interested nowadays in simplified ideas about punishment and "getting tough" as the "newly discovered answer" to crime and delinquency. Yet it was not really that long ago that Bill Lewis was recruited by the California Youth Authority to do the work he describes in this book because "getting tough" was not working in correctional facilities. Perhaps the pendulum is now swinging again. Bill's book provides fuel to a renaissance.

I commend this book to those interested in integrating ideas of therapeutic intervention into the manner in which delinquent youths are treated. As a textbook, it will be excellent for the classroom because of its heavy emphasis on the application of theory through actual case studies. The information that the book provides can be useful as a guide to the creation of a treatment modality within any correctional environment. Should a correctional administrator wish to change his program into a "treatment program," the ingredients are here. Bill outlines the prerequisites for such an environment as well as a process for its implementation.

I had not read Bill Lewis's writings for several years, until I read this book. It was a pleasure to see that he has not lost his knack of being able to present complex ideas in simple, everyday language that we can all understand. One of Bill's greatest contributions at Paso Robles was his entertaining and plain-speaking written material. The Superintendent, Gerald Spencer, used Bill's writings as one of his major resources in communicating to line staff as his administration implemented treatment programs. The case histories he wrote for us then were always more like interesting prose than the boring case studies, full of "in-house" psychological verbiage, that I was used to reading from the "typical" psychologist. Bill's stories are still well worth reading for the pure, human enjoyment of reading.

So if you are not going to school, if you are not a correctional worker seeking knowledge, and you are not a correctional administrator trying to improve your program—then just read Bill's book because, if the subject matter interests you, you cannot help but find reading this book an enjoyable experience. Enjoy!

Loren W. Look
Consultant in Criminal Justice

Introduction

What is this book? Is it a training manual for group-living supervisors? Is it a guide for parents trying to do their best at raising their kids? Is it a textbook to give college criminal justice majors a glimpse at what really awaits them out there? Is it a source of ideas for therapists beclouded by university brainwashing and seeking better ways to help people? Is it a history of the treatment programs that now exist in *every* institution in the California Youth Authority, others across the U.S.A., and some around the world? Is it a segment of the author's autobiography?

The answer is yes. It is all of these.

I have attempted to convey a frame of reference regarding how personalities develop (and maldevelop). From this perspective, some logical implications for corrective treatment are identified. Techniques for implementing this treatment are then described and illustrated.

The personality requirements and interpersonal skills of an effective youth counselor are defined. A self-administered quiz, scoring instructions, and discussion of each item are presented. This quiz permits current and potential youth workers to evaluate their own interpersonal styles in terms of youthwork effectiveness. It is also an excellent training device that has been used in correctional science classes as well as in-service training programs.

Milieu therapy in group living programs is explained and illustrated in an historical account of the development of the California Youth Authority's first treatment program for emotionally disturbed offenders.

Definition and discussion of personality counseling are followed by instruction in specific individual and group therapy techniques. These are illustrated from actual case files. Included are two uncommon and effective approaches that I have come to call "Why Not?" therapy and "Behind the Back" small group therapy. The use of drawing, weight-lifting, tape recording, and other adjuncts to verbal approaches are discussed.

The book concludes with a "how to" discussion of a large-group method — "Community Counseling" — and a brief tribute to some of the people who have unwittingly contributed to my eclectic frame of reference.

A special thank you goes to Buell E. Goocher, Executive Director of the Boys and Girls Mental Health Centers, a broad-based child and youth services agency in the San Diego area. Dr. Goocher's editorial suggestions were of inestimable value in helping me smooth out rough spots and apply the final coat of polish.

I have tried to provide, in fun-to-read form, training material for youthworkers, thought-provoking ideas for therapists, useful mental health and child-rearing principles for parents, and information that can help the ordinary guy on the street better understand some of his oddball neighbors and their kids (and perhaps his own, as well).

Chapter 1

Sizing Up Delinquents' Heads

To my juvenile delinquent clientele, I am known as a head-shrinker. Headshrinking, sometimes called psychotherapy, actually involves no shrinking of heads.[1] What it does involve is a special kind of relationship between two people which permits the one (the headshrinker) to employ certain techniques acquired in his training to help the other (the shrinkee, more specific to this book, the juvenile delinquent).

These methods can help the shrinkee to assume greater self-responsibility, to clarify and resolve troublesome feelings, to gain self-understanding, to think more clearly, to get along better with other people, to derive more satisfaction from life, and to cope more effectively with problems and frustrations. Now that we have a rough idea of what headshrinking aims to do, let us examine the shrinkee. What is the juvenile delinquent? That should be easy to answer. But is it?

A juvenile delinquent, according to one school of thought, is a minor who is guilty of an act which would make him a criminal if he were an adult. This is not an entirely correct assumption. There are a number of "delinquents" in our institutions who were committed for acts which are socially acceptable and commonplace among adults, such as possessing alcohol or participating in sexual relations by mutual consent.[2]

Another definition might be that a juvenile delinquent is anyone committed to an institution for juvenile delinquents. If so, we exclude the juveniles who indulge in robberies, assaults, mayhem, and other such diversions without being caught. (Oh yes, there are some.) Are they not delinquents?

A droll, if equally incomplete, concept is that a delinquent is an adolescent who does today what we did at his age. The universality of the term, "we" in this definition is questionable. Police services are more abundant and effective now than when "we" engaged in sit-ins and reassembled the VW Bug on top of the college administration building; and there are some juveniles now in institutions for having committed very similar atrocities. However, there are also some who committed armed robbery, rape and murder who persuade me not to define the juvenile delinquent in terms of what "I" did as a youngster.

We seem to be making negligible progress toward defining "The Juvenile Delinquent." Perhaps there is no such single entity. As a matter of fact, there isn't. There are a lot of different kinds.

Juvenile delinquents are people. Basically, they are not very different from other people. They need the same things that you and I need. The only difference is that you and I had those things given to us, or learned how to get them in ways that did not bring the wrath of society down upon us. Juvenile delinquents, due to no choice of their own, are born into situations where they are not given enough of those things, and are not taught acceptable ways of getting them. Since some of the things they need are essential to continued human existence, they must invent ways of getting them, even at the expense of invoking society's anger, or crawl into a hole and die. Which would you do?

What are these things they must have for survival? Ice cream? Cars? Swimming pools? No. These are not basic human needs. In addition to the essential physical needs for air, water, food, and shelter, there are certain inborn psychological needs which must be satisfied minimally if infant human beings are to continue living at all, and must be satisfied abundantly if they are to grow into normal, healthy adult personalities. One of these is love.[3] Another is consistency and predictability in the way people respond. Still another requires that limits or controls be set to prevent infants from hurting themselves or getting the idea that the rest of the world exists only to satisfy their whims. The need for new experience is yet another.

The degree to, and conditions under, which these needs are satisfied (or frustrated) in childhood, play a major role in determining the kind of adult personality which eventually emerges.

It would be impossible for me to describe completely the combination of needs, satisfactions, and frustrations which go into the making of just one personality. Instead of attempting this, let us just take a closer look at two of these basic psychological needs, (1) the need for love and (2) the need for limits or external control, and see how they interact and influence the development of personality.

We can represent love satisfaction by a horizontal line, and external control by a vertical line, as in Figure 1.

The plus end of the line indicates maximal satisfaction of the need. The minus end of the line represents minimal satisfaction. Now, using this model, we can point out a few cause and effect relationships.

First, what is the ideal situation? What combination of these two ingredients is the recipe for normal, healthy adulthood? The formula: a full measure of love throughout the growth period, blended with a diminishing quantity of external control.

When babies are born they must have complete control and protection to survive. As they mature they become more and more capable of controlling and protecting themselves. As adults, hopefully, they can stand on their own two feet as independent, self-controlled citizens. (See Figure 2.) Now, for the benefit of parents

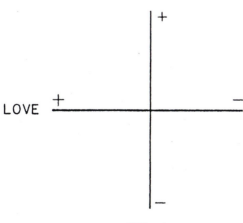

EXTERNAL CONTROL

FIG. I

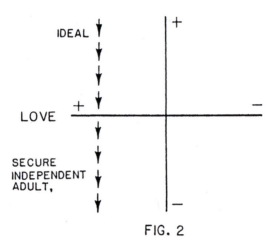

FIG. 2

who have a flair for the different, or who are interested in pre-selecting a certain kind of personality deviation for their children, let us try out a few other love-control combinations on our model.

Suppose the children receive *maximal love* along with *maximal control which is maintained as they mature.* They are not allowed to make decisions, take chances, or venture forth into the world. Consequently, they never learn how to do these things intelligently. They grow up to be helpless oafs who are at a complete loss as to how to deal with the world when circumstance at last separates them from their loving protectors. They are the *overprotected children* who become the overdependent adults. (See Figure 3.) They may be found on welfare, skid row, drifting, or in mental hospitals.

What happens if the children receive *maximal love* along with *minimal control?* They learn to take, but not to give. Anything their little hearts desire is theirs. Anything they wish to do they do, as their doting parents beam.

They begin to surmise that they are something pretty special. They do not develop a sensitivity to the needs and rights of others, since others make no demands upon their behavior.

They are rudely shocked by school teachers, and later by employers, who insist that they really are mortal and must work for what they receive. Our scientific name for them is *spoiled brats*. (See Figure 4.)

Now we come to our first unloved child. How does *minimal love* combine with *overcontrol*? First, the child, feeling the lack of love,

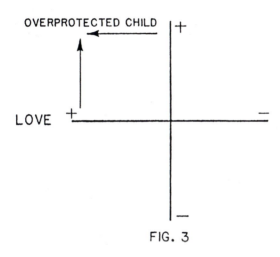

FIG. 3

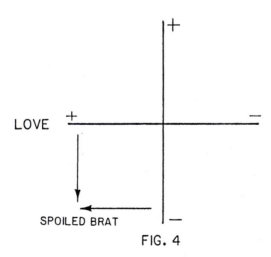

FIG. 4

responds appropriately by disliking the parents and wanting to rebel against their demands. These rejecting parents, however, have adopted the philosophy that since they are stuck with the unwanted child, they will take the course of least potential trouble, which they perceive to be to hold it still, keep it shut up, and out of their hair.

This child is not allowed to have opinions or feelings, to make decisions, or to explore the world. It is spoken to only in harsh, demanding tones. It attempts to rebel against this physical and emotional binding, for despite the parents' efforts to remain unaware of it, the child really is a human being with all the basic needs of the race.

These children learn quickly that they cannot rebel. They are no match for their giant captors. After a few feeble attempts to gain freedom, earning nothing but a beating for their efforts, they give up. Their spirit is broken.

They sneak, slink, avoid speaking when possible, and try to live in the shadows of life, so that no one will notice them. They are sure that if they are noticed, people will harm them.

As they grow up, they offer themselves as doormats for everyone's feet. They cannot defend their rights against anyone. They are especially afraid of adults.

If they are boys, as their sexual impulses grow stronger, they may molest children in a feeble attempt to satisfy their own needs without risking the rejection or anger of a grown-up woman. Girls may become sexual pushovers, unable to assert their rights by saying no.

They see themselves as low, unlovable, cowardly, inferior, worthless, creatures in the midst of a threatening, cruel world which hates them. They sometimes wonder who they are and what they are doing in the world at all. They are *cowed personalities*. (See Figure 5.)

There is one more possible combination of the extreme poles on our model. That is *minimal love* with *minimal control*. Here, as with the cowed personality the parents do not want the child. These parents, however, elect the course of least resistance in dealing with the situation. Beyond half-heartedly and unreliably providing food, water and shelter, they ignore him. (Arbitrarily, this child is a boy, as were most of the youths in the author's clinical experience.)

EXTERNAL CONTROL

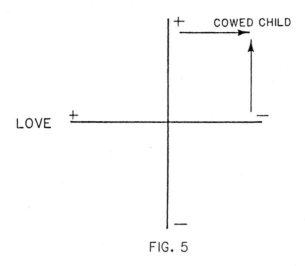

FIG. 5

From the lack of love, he feels dissatisfied and lonely. He also feels anger toward the parents who do not give him the warmth and acceptance he sees other children receiving from their parents. Gradually his anger spreads to cover all people in authority — teachers, policemen and adults in general.

Armed with two burning emotions, the need for love and bitter anger toward the adult world which treats him as a nobody, he suddenly becomes aware that his parents (if he has two by this time) don't especially care whether he comes or goes. He goes. He goes down the back streets and alleys at any time of day or night. He encounters some other fellows about his own age down on the corner. He is attracted to them. They seem to understand. They offer him an opportunity. If he will break the window out of the police station, proving that he really is a kindred soul and not a chicken, they will give him the love, acceptance and respect which he craves so deeply. Does he hesitate? Huh! It isn't every day that a fellow gets a chance to express his anger and be accepted as a person all at once.

Compared with his past life, he is now a success. Life has some meaning for the first time. At last he is somebody. He is an *aggressive delinquent*. (See Figure 6.)

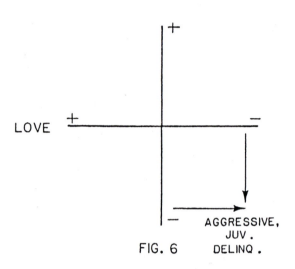

EXTERNAL CONTROL

LOVE

FIG. 6

AGGRESSIVE,
JUV .
DELINQ .

NOTES

1. Nor any other body parts, for that matter.

2. I use the term "socially acceptable" here to signify what society *does*, not what it says people should do. We are a hypocritical lot whose behavior in private is frequently quite different from what we, as a society, publicly profess that it should be.

3. You don't believe that love is really that important to life? Run down to the library and look up the literature on *marasmus*. This is a disease of infancy, related to extreme deprivation of love. Its symptoms are progressive apathy, loss of appetite and eventual death.

Chapter II

Some Heads Are Sanforized

We older generation protesters, sit-in participants, and Bug reassemblers were *adaptive*, or *cultural*, delinquents. This is the best kind to be if it is in fact the "best" to be any kind of delinquent at all. We were happy, had friends, were accepted by them, and enjoyed sharing certain recreational activities with them. We adapted successfully to the subculture to which we belonged.

The only fly in the ointment was that, in the eyes of the larger society, our whole subculture was delinquent.

About half of our institutionalized delinquents today are of a similar breed. Some modern adolescent subcultures enjoy such recreations as drug parties, shooting guns from passing cars, and painting *placas* on other people's property. But these people still get along with each other, are self-accepting, and, in general, are a pretty happy and well-adjusted lot in their own circles.

Adaptive delinquents, without benefit of headshrinking, tend to grow up, get married, shed the social values of their teenage subcultures, and adopt those of adult society, of which they are automatically made members by the process of maturation.

Intensive headshrinking would not be a very practical approach to cultural delinquency. There are overwhelmingly too many stinkers for the number of shrinkers. All of the professional psychotherapists in the country, in a concentrated attack, could barely scratch the surface of the cultural delinquent population.

Furthermore, the adaptive delinquent's head is sanforized. It is pre-shrunk, and all right the way it is. Remember that within himself, and within his subculture, he is a pretty adequate fellow who can satisfy his own social and emotional needs and otherwise successfully cope with life and its problems.

Headshrinking is designed primarily for people who are un-happy, deficient in the ability to satisfy their needs, and incapable of satisfactorily adjusting to life and its problems.

Does this mean that cultural delinquency is not a real problem? It does not. The problem is very real and very costly. Headshrinking simply is not the weapon of choice to combat it.

What methods, then, might be effective in combatting cultural delinquency? Since the problem, in essence, consists of unaccepta-ble (to us) behavior which is permitted, or even encouraged, by certain groups, gangs, or even whole neighborhoods, efforts toward solution might logically be directed toward these groups, rather than individuals. In attempting to persuade a delinquent subculture to abandon its offensive behaviors and values, two general ap-proaches are possible. (1) Force the members, by threat of punish-ment, to conform to our standards. (2) Expose them to socially acceptable experiences which are basically more satisfying than their antisocial activities which we wish to see abolished.

The first approach, a show of force by police, may be expedient at times, as in an emergency situation created by two rival gangs squaring off for a rumble with tire chains, switchblades, and zip-guns.

As a long-range solution to cultural delinquency, however, the famous "get tough" policy is self-defeating in two ways.

First, it is doomed to failure economically. Rule by threat and force, by its nature a challenge and an invitation to rebellion, de-mands increasing numbers of policemen, weapons, and punishment facilities. The cost of enforcement comes to exceed the cost of the damages which would have occurred in the absence of the effort.

Second, rule by threat and force is self-defeating in that it em-bodies the very values which we hope to persuade these gang-ori-ented adolescents to abandon in favor of mature social courtesy and cooperation. Why should *they* abandon these tactics in human rela-tions when the society trying to motivate them to do so, uses them?

Juveniles sometimes have difficulty in making clear distinctions between the moral implications of being knocked on the head with a tire chain or with a policeman's club. If we (society, including po-licemen) really want to persuade delinquent subcultures to abandon certain behaviors and do things our way, an essential step is to examine ourselves critically and make sure that "our way" really is different or better from theirs, or more desirable, or more likely to elicit the applause of the social environment.

The second general approach to cultural delinquency exposes the culprit groups to socially acceptable experiences which provide greater need satisfaction than do their delinquencies. This offers far greater promise of a long-term solution than does the "get tough" paradox. This has been demonstrated in a number of communities by social group workers, agencies and citizens organizations, providing legitimate channels for status-gaining, financial achievement, recreation, and social interaction to members of delinquent subcultures.

Since half of the juvenile institutional population consists of cultural delinquents, and since psychotherapy is an inappropriate approach to this group, what, if anything, can be done? Basically, the treatment of cultural delinquents in institutions employs the same principles that work in the outside community. *Milieu*, or environment, therapy consists of providing the inmates with a daily living program in which they can experience achievement, respect, warmth, understanding, external controls appropriate to their level of self-responsibility, and democratic leadership.[1] They learn, through experiencing, the gratifications afforded by civilized cooperative living. Unfortunately, upon leaving the institution, they often return to their own delinquent subcultures and find that what they have learned in the institution about human relations cannot be applied in the home neighborhood. Though prepared for a more mature and satisfying style of life, they cannot have it, unless community treatment is applied to their subculture, or until age permits them to escape into a vocation and marriage.

NOTE

1. It would be amusing if it were not so tragic that some influential people believe that exposure to a harsh, punitive, dictatorship within an institution is a good way to prepare inmates for successful living in the democratic society to which they will return.

Chapter III

"Headshrinking":
Who Needs It?

It is the other fifty percent—the maladaptive delinquents—to whom the headshrinker in a correctional setting addresses himself. *Who are* these youngsters who need the services of the headshrinker? This question contains more than meets the eye—namely, its own answer. Those delinquents who need therapy are those *who do not know who they are.*

Maybe *we* know who they are, or can find out by studying their social histories, but *they* don't know. "Headshrinking" with delinquents consists largely of helping *them* to find out. None of us know who we are when we first come into the world. We are little bundles of raw needs, and only gradually come to recognize ourselves as persons. The kind of persons we eventually see ourselves to be depends, in addition to imprecisely understood physiological, biochemical and genetic factors, upon how the world (people) treats us (satisfies our needs) as we are searching for our identities. If the world treats us with love, we can say to ourselves, "Aha! That is who I am! I am someone nice; someone good; someone worthy of being loved." If, during those early years, we have met active rejection, we have another answer to our question of identity: "I am someone unloveable; someone bad; someone deserving of loathing and disrespect." If we are largely ignored—treated in not much of any way at all—we cannot learn much about who we are. We can only conclude, "I must be nobody at all."

Hopefully, each person, as he matures, receives satisfying treatment from the world in an ever increasing variety of situations. He needs to learn who he is in relation to many segments of the world, and at many levels of intimacy. If asked, "Who are you?" the well-developed adolescent personality could perhaps reply, "I am Joe Jones, my parents' son, my girlfriend's steady, a senior in high school, a member of the swimming team, a Methodist, and a Young Democrat."*

Ask yourself who *you* are, and respond with the first five answers that come to mind. If you are a reasonably well-balanced adult, you should be able to identify yourself quickly at several levels of abstraction — as a participating member of several different sized units of the world, such as Joe Jones did in the preceding paragraph.

How do you imagine maladaptive delinquents reply to that same question? Let's ask some and find out.[2] The question, "Will you give me now, at least four answers to this question: Who are you? Just whatever comes to mind." (Names are changed.)

Delinquent A.

1. James Albert Jordon
2. A Negro
3. I have grey eyes
4. Can't think of nothing else

Delinquent B.

1. Frank Gonzales
2. Father is (name)
3. Mother is (name)
4. Brother is (name)
5. Other brother is (name)
6. Sister is (name)

Delinquent C.

1. Robert Fife
2. Can't think of no more
3. — — —
4. — — —

---

*Or possibly even a Young Republican.

Delinquent D.

1. I'm a boy
2. Kenneth Hodson
3. Male species
4. Of masculine sex

Delinquent E.
1. Leon Stott
2. Boy
3. Human being
4. Something living

Delinquent F.
1. A human
2. My name is Phinney
3. I'm 15
4. I'm going to school in the YA (Youth Authority)

Delinquent G.
1. A boy
2. I'm also Harold Kelley
3. Animal
4. Person

Delinquent H.
1. Chris Nichols
2. Age 18
3. Height 5' 11"
4. Male sex

Delinquent I.
1. Me
2. Harry Turner
3. Myself
4. and I

Delinquent J.
1. Human being
2. A person
3. An animal
4. Nothing else

Note that, while the delinquent boys (usually) can meet the basic request for four answers, that the *range* of units of the world with which each boy can identify himself is extremely limited. Frank Gonzales, in six answers, identifies himself only as an individual who is related to each member of his immediate family. Kenneth Hodson seems to know only that he has a name and is male. Leon Stott, Harold Kelley and J. see themselves merely as vague members of vague masses (persons, humans, boys, living creatures, etc.). Robert Fife and Harry Turner cannot go beyond naming themselves, apparently lacking feelings of identification with any units of the world outside themselves.

"Headshrinking," who needs it? Nobody in this group. "Headshrinking" is probably the most inappropriate, inaccurate nickname anyone possibly could have dreamed up for what these boys really need. There is nothing swollen here that requires shrinking. These are normal sized human personality shells, which are dismally, dreadfully empty. What these heads need is filling, not shrinking.

NOTE

1. These are the actual replies to the "Who are you?" question given by several institutionalized delinquent boys in their mid-teens, selected randomly from the writer's case files.

Chapter IV

How Empty Heads Are Stuffed

Many maladaptive delinquents cannot profit from headshrinking in its classic sense—soaring back to early childhood on a couch, searching for infantile experiences which frightened them into behaving neurotically. This approach is better suited to wealthy folks in Beverly Hills seeking high fashion (and equally high priced) professional absolution for their sins.

In fact, delinquents who come into contact with classical, analytic therapists frequently wind up in worse shape than when they started. One reason is that many of them do not have sufficiently developed personalities to permit them to understand what the hell this therapist is talking about—what it is he expects them to do, or to understand about themselves. Since these unsophisticated fellows can't grasp the object of the game (recall forgotten traumata and "gain insight" into their effects on current behavior), their therapists get annoyed at them for being so stupid, and reject them.¹

Thus, the delinquent, already suffering from a poor sense of identity and low self-esteem, gets cut down yet another notch.

Those maladaptive delinquents who *can* grasp the analysis game more often than not use it to rationalize their antisocial behavior, rather than to rectify it. "Oh, so I steal cars because my mother caught me masturbating and took away my pogo stick? Well, then, the car stealing is my *mother's* fault, isn't it? So, I can go ahead and do it without feeling guilty, right?"

There are *some* individual delinquents for whom a bit of classical type headshrinking, especially in combination with much headfilling (ego building), can do some good. But a great number of delinquent youths simply have underdeveloped, partially empty heads which need filling, not shrinking.[2] Let's take another look at how personalities develop, and see why this is true.

Recall that the newborn's personality is largely a bundle of needs — physical and emotional. During the early months of life, the infant is totally dependent upon elders to satisfy those needs. Its very life is in the hands of the parents or other care givers. The infant's *total* personality at this stage, if one could draw personalities, might look like this:

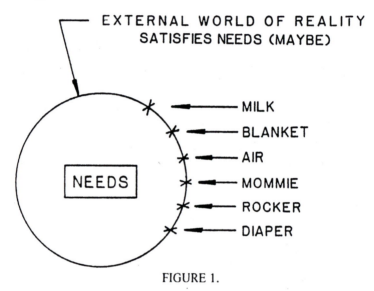

EXTERNAL WORLD OF REALITY
SATISFIES NEEDS (MAYBE)

NEEDS

MILK
BLANKET
AIR
MOMMIE
ROCKER
DIAPER

FIGURE 1.

But where does it go from there? And how does it get there? Let's jump ahead twenty years and check the situation.

The basic need system with which this infant began life still forms the core of his personality as a young man. By this time these needs have branched out and assumed many forms at many levels of abstraction. For example, the need for love may now be satisfied through such diverse experiences as recognition for achievement, concern, sympathy, applause, or sexual union.

In addition to this increased complexity within his need system itself, we note that our young adult's perceived world of external reality has become vastly more complicated. No longer consisting entirely of Mommy and Daddy, the external world has become a

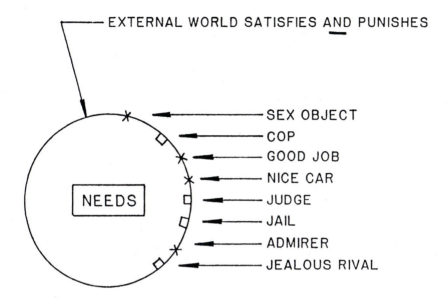

FIGURE 2.

garden of choices — a veritable supermarket of persons and objects which can be employed to satisfy his needs. What a glorious position to be in — the hungry child turned loose in the candy shop — except for one complication (actually, two, as we will see in a moment). In addition to all those neat, need-gratifying goodies, the external world of reality is infested with rules, or laws, governing the conditions under which people may *and may not* satisfy their needs. Along with these rules come cops, judges, jailers, bosses who fire people, irate shopkeepers, and jealous spouses, all waiting to pounce on and punish anyone who gets caught satisfying his needs at unapproved times and places, in inappropriate ways, or with unauthorized persons and objects. It becomes apparent that our young adult could not survive in the real world if his personality consisted solely of a bigger and better need system. Every time a need cried out for gratification, he would grasp the first good looking object that appeared on the horizon and gratify away, nine times out of ten getting himself jailed or shot in the process.* In order for our young man to have reached age twenty in freedom and health, he *must* have developed another personality component along the way. He did. Freud called it the *ego*.

"Ego" has become an everyday word in the American vocabulary, used casually, frequently, and most often, incorrectly. There really isn't such a thing. No one has ever seen an ego.** It is simply a theoretical construct — a complex image synthesized in, and by, men's minds to explain men's minds. Much scholarly prose has been written about the functions of the ego. Detailed review is not necessary for our purposes.

At the moment we are concerned with the survival and freedom of our hypothetical young adult. He needs *something* to act as a buffer and arbitrator between that demanding need system of his and the regulations and threatened punishments of the external world of reality. We'll just add this component to his personality picture and call it an ego.

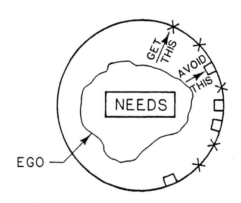

X = NEED SATISFYING OBJECT

□ = PENALTY

FIGURE 3.

---

*And the process is a tender and painful place to be shot.

**A fact which will not stop me from drawing one a few moments from now.

Now with an intact and properly functioning ego*, our twenty-year-old should be able to get along fine. At this stage, the ego's job is twofold. It must (1) *obtain* need satisfaction for our young man under conditions which (2) keep him from coming into conflict with society's rules and regulations.

Ego failure in function (1), obtaining need satisfaction, is associated with neurotic unhappiness — chronic frustration.

Ego failure in function (2), testing and avoiding conflict with social rules, is a major source of irresponsible, delinquent behavior.

A second complication (other than society's rules and punishments) interferes with the need system's attempted adjustment to reality. In addition to "growing" an ego, the maturing young person also "grows" a set of personal values — his *own* rules and regulations governing how he may or may not satisfy his needs, *and* his own self-punishing system — a conscience.[3]

While the conscience has no direct power to control behavior (either give rise to or prohibit need gratification), it has the power to punish its owner *after* he has violated his own inner code. It can make him ache with guilt, and blindly enter into ineffective self-punishing activities (self-degradation, clumsy lawbreaking aimed at getting himself caught and punished, attempted suicide, etc.). Thus the presence of the conscience adds another dimension to the ego's job. The ego (which can and does directly give rise to, or prohibit, need-gratifying acts) must now (1) *obtain* need satisfaction while (2) avoiding conflict with society's sanctions and (3) avoiding violation of conscience and consequent self-punishment.

Now our hypothetical twenty-year-old is really cooking on all burners. His intact, properly functioning ego is seeing to it that his needs are satisfied, that his relationship with external reality is harmonious and that he is at peace with himself — consistently abiding by his own set of inner values. How did he get here? Where did that ego and set of personal inner values come from? What went on between birth and age twenty that brought all this to pass?

Recall once again that the newborn infant is primarily a bundle of needs, both physical and emotional. If *totally* deprived of need grat-

---

*Aren't you glad you finally got to see one? Looks like a fried egg, doesn't it? Ego or eggo — what's the difference?

ification, the baby dies. If his physical needs are perfectly met, his body grows and matures until it assumes strong, healthy adult proportions. If his emotional needs are perfectly met, his personality will evolve from a mere primitive need system into the strong, healthy adult personality ascribed to our young man in the preceding paragraph.[4]

The ego and personal value system come into existence through a process variously called "identification," "internalization," or "absorption." The one who is doing the emotional nourishing becomes an ego model to the nourished one. The infant gradually *absorbs* or *internalizes* portions of the personalities and characters of the mother, the father, and significant others along the way who provide need gratification. This *identification* with the emotional nourishment-givers takes place unconsciously. Its end result, after years of sorting, shuffling, integration and reintegration of traits, characteristics and values, is a unique organization of these borrowed and internalized components. It is a personality which resembles those of its primary contributors in some ways, but is, in fact, one of a kind—different from any other personality on earth.

So it is, during the period from birth to adulthood, some empty heads are pretty well filled with egos and values. Others are not. Delinquents tend to grow up with only partially filled heads. Their egos are fragmented—full of holes—which permits a large number of their impulses for need gratification to be discharged directly and irrationally onto the outside world without benefit of foresight or regard for consequences.

We now know a few things about maladaptive delinquents which ought to have some implications as to what we will have to do if we are to "habilitate" them.

We know that they *don't know* who they are, except in very limited ways. They live in small worlds of experience, have impoverished senses of identity, and often search for meaning in life and a sense of being *someone* through antisocial behavior. Thus, the would-be "habilitator" is going to have to discover or devise, ways to help them *find out* who they are—broaden their worlds of social experience.

We also know that the portions of their personalities responsible

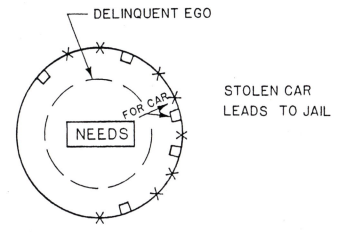

NEED SHOOTS THROUGH HOLES.
IMPULSIVENESS LEADS TO PENALTY.

FIGURE 4.

for gaining need satisfaction while avoiding conflict with the laws and punishments are not fully developed. Their egos are riddled with great gaps, either because their emotional needs were not adequately met as they grew up, or else their needs *were* adequately met, but by lousy ego models.[5] The treatment implication here is that those ego holes need to be patched.

How do we do these things — teach people who they are and patch holes in egos? That's what the rest of this book is about.

NOTES

1. Either by labeling them "unsuitable" and terminating therapy, or by continuing "treatment" sarcastically and condescendingly, depending on how the fees are coming in. (Have you ever noticed what becomes of the word "therapist" if you separate it between the e and the r?)

2. Another way to put this is that delinquents can't be rehabilitated, because they never were habilitated in the first place. You can't repair something that doesn't yet exist.

3. Or "superego," if you want to be fancy and Freudian.

4. It should be pointed out that no such perfection exists in the personality and character of mortal man. Everyone's ego at times fails to do its job, producing frustration, antisocial behavior, and guilt feelings. The average man probably owes a couple of years in prison if all the facts were known. Some of us more.

5. For example, the youth who received adequate love, control, consistency, etc., but from a father who spends most of his time in jail and a streetwalking mother.

Chapter V

Patching Egos —
General Principles

As far as I know, there is only one basic way to fill the holes in a poorly developed ego. That is to employ, by design, the same forces that spontaneously produce healthy egos in those who are blessed with them. Correctional staff, volunteers, and even delinquent peers under positive conditions, can "rub off" favorably on the underdeveloped, fragmented personality of a delinquent youth.

The staff member, by gratifying the legitimate human needs of the youth, *becomes* an ego model with whom the delinquent begins to identify. *If his needs are being satisfied*, the youth, over a period of time, unconsciously absorbs portions of the staff member's personality — values as well as ego strengths — and adopts them as his own. The staff member's personality provides transfusions of ego strength which are integrated with the delinquent's personality structure, shoring up weakness and filling gaps.

Remember, identification is largely an *unconscious* process, and may *not* be brought about directly through punishment, preaching, bribery, or coercion. These practices, unfortunately too often relied upon by correctional workers, can produce changes in surface behavior — superficial compliance or conformity. But these changes are fake. They do not reflect real absorption of new strengths and values, and they disappear as soon as the external pressure is removed.

Genuine personality growth — the incorporation of new strengths and values into the delinquent's *self*, so they become part of him — takes place only through the unconscious absorption of these characteristics from a donor — someone who meets his legitimate human needs (such as love, control, consistency, new experience and their derivatives).

Of course, in the correctional treatment setting, the worker (ego model) should not attempt to gratify his clients' needs at the same level of abstraction at which they should have been satisfied by parents in the first place.[1] Instead, he must sharpen his skill at looking behind behavior to find out what basic human needs are being expressed, and develop methods for gratifying them in ways that are appropriate to the client's maturity level. A correctional worker can meet the need for love, for example, at the young adult level through such means as courtesy; showing genuine interest and concern; giving instructions in a friendly, respectful way (as opposed to grumpy or profane barking); giving honest praise for work well done; and asking for opinions and respecting them as worthwhile. The correctional worker, be he classroom teacher, houseparent, counselor, guard, coach, or trade instructor, who gives love to his clients in these ways becomes an ego model. Not only is he meeting the legitimate human need for love, but this *same* behavior may well satisfy some of the delinquent youth's *other* basic socio-emotional needs. Such treatment may well be a *new experience* for a youth who has in the past experienced only rejection and discourtesy from adults. *Consistency* in such treatment permits necessary *control* to be maintained with a minimum of conflict and resistance. Respect earns respect. Threats and coercive control earn fear, hatred, and (perhaps) grudging temporary conformity.

Thus, consistent treatment of the delinquent youth with love (which means with dignity and necessary firmness — not mollycoddling or laxness), establishes the worker as an ego model, and the hole-patching operation is under way. But it does much more than that!

Remember our other goal — helping the delinquent youth to find out who he is — to develop in him a broader and more satisfying sense of identity. How do people find out who they are? How do they develop a self-concept? Through other people's responses to them. The infant whose parents ignore or abuse him develops a view of himself as someone worthy only of rejection and abuse. Later, a correctional worker treating him consistently with love challenges the validity of this poor self-image. "How come he treats me so good if I'm all that bad?'' The unfortunate youth, at this point, will often put the worker to the test—do things designed to make the worker blow his cool and reject him. Being treated as a "good" person is pleasant and exciting, but it is also confusing and scary to one who has long viewed himself as bad and unworthy of such treatment. "What's this guy up to? He couldn't really like me. He must be running a game on me to get something or hurt me in the long run. I'd better not fall for it. I'll show him what a nasty guy I really am. That'll turn him off.'' Selfchange, even in the direction of improvement, is frightening, carrying with it the spectre of possible failure and destruction of the self in a new, unfamiliar role.

If the correctional worker is mature and understands this conflict generated in his client by the love treatment, he will be patient with the youth's tantrums, or whatever obnoxious tricks he pulls to try to bring about rejection by the worker in order to preserve his lousy, but safely familiar, self-image. The worker will firmly, but kindly, set reasonable limits upon the youngster's antisocial stunts, but will *never* take the bait and respond in kind with viciousness, ego-deflating sarcasm, aloofness, or any of those behaviors that communicate personal dislike and rejection.

If the worker *continues, continues,* and *continues* to give love, external control and consistency in the face of his client's attempts to bring on rejection, eventually the old, rotten self-image will be forced to change. It will have been *proved* invalid. The youngster will have no choice but to conclude, "Hey! I couldn't be all bad. This guy really likes me and cares about me. Therefore, I must be worthy of being liked and cared about, at least in this relationship. If I'm a worthwhile person to him, maybe I could be to others too. If he likes me, he is my friend. If he is my friend, I am his friend. Hey, Man! Fantastic! I know who I am! I am a friend.''

It is truly one of life's most beautiful experiences to take a hand in producing such a transformation. The miserable, frightened, self-condemned, shadow-dwelling misfit steps out into the sunlight and begins to walk with head erect, a smile on his face, savoring his first taste of a delicious, brand new experience—the feeling of being a worthwhile human being.

Psychiatric training or a degree in psychology or social work is not necessary to perform this kind of marvelous service.[2] Good parents do it right from the start. Any warm, sensitive, rational and caring human being can learn to identify other's legitimate needs and to gratify them. Some folks have personalities which permit them to meet other's needs automatically and constantly. These are the people we enjoy being around, and when we are around them, some of their personalities "rub off" on us. We identify with them.

This information should tell us something about who ought to be working with delinquent youths, and who *shouldn't*. The two primary requirements are that youth workers *must* have the sensitivity and maturity to identify and meet the needs of others in their everyday interactions, whatever they may be, and they *must* themselves have healthy, well-developed egos and value systems, so that they may serve as *effective* models. Given these two assets as a starting point, ongoing training in special techniques will produce limitless increase in human relations skill and effectiveness. Lacking these two characteristics, all the formal training and professional status symbols (degrees) in the world will be to no avail.

Now, let's find out what kind of an ego model *you* are, or would be if you chose to work with troubled youth.

NOTES

1. For example, very few seventeen-year-old gangfighters respond positively to being cuddled lovingly and rocked in a rocking chair by a correctional officer.

2. In fact, there are some such specialists who can't do it at all, either because they personally never had much love-giving capacity, or have become vain and dehumanized through worship of their own "professional" status.

Chapter VI

Would You Be a Good Ego Model?
Let's Find Out

In an institution, camp, group home, or other such facility, a variety of specific interpersonal and intragroup treatment techniques may be deployed by professional ego patchers.* The trouble is that none of them work unless they are applied in a setting which supports them.

Who do you think has the most effect on an institutionalized delinquent youth's attitudes, behavior and personality growth — the learned psychologist who lays wise counsel and exotic therapies on him for forty minutes a week? Wrong! It is the houseparent who spends forty *hours* per week with the youth. Or the teacher who works with him six hours a day in the classroom. Or the crew boss teaching him how to clear firebreaks in the forest all day. Or, perhaps most of all, the other delinquent youths in the program.[1]

These key figures in the youth's everyday, elbow-rubbing, interpersonal environment will largely determine whether his personality is strengthened, left as is, or further damaged by the experience. They are the ones who meet his needs — or frustrate them — day in and day out. They are the ones whose values, character and interpersonal behaviors the delinquent is likely to try on for size, experiment with, and adopt as his own if they prove effective and satisfying. How good would you be as a youth leader? Would you have the sensitivity to recognize the basic emotional needs underlying a delinquent's** interpersonal behavior? If you are sensitive to his needs, is your own everyday interpersonal behavior skillful enough

---

*We will explore some of these techniques in detail later.
**Or anybody's, for that matter.

to meet those needs? If so, how good is your own ability to test reality, make wise judgments, and stay out of trouble while enjoying life (satisfying your own needs)? Should you be able to meet the delinquent youth's needs, causing him to identify with you—absorb and adopt portions of your personality and values—would the results be a significant improvement, or would our youth turn out to be more fragmented, or a worse crook, than when you met him? Would you be worth a damn as an ego model? Let's give you a quiz and find out.

This self-scoring quiz is not concerned with your knowledge of special subject matter or your proficiency at any specific trade or profession. Rather, it is aimed at exploring your attitudes toward your fellow human beings as reflected in the ways you would behave toward them as a leader (or ego model). Whether your specific job might be teaching delinquent youths arithmetic, how to mow lawns, or seeing to it that they shower and brush their teeth, your most important impact upon them will *not* be in *what* you teach them or do with them, but in *the way you go about it*—your style as a human being relating to them as human beings.

Scoring instructions will follow the quiz. Your score may suggest to you whether, as a worker with delinquent youth, you would most likely function as a truly growth-inspiring leader and ego model; as a neutral, more or less harmless caretaker; or as a destructive influence, inflicting further damage on these young personalities whose development already has been stunted and distorted.

Be truthful with yourself. Imagine yourself on the job as a supervisor of delinquent youths. Check the answer on each item[2] which seems to best fit you. If you aren't sure, guess.

SO YOU'RE A YOUTH LEADER?—
A QUIZ

1. I punish the whole group in my care, or several of its members, for the misbehavior of an individual.
   A. Often_____ B. Sometimes_____
   C. Rarely or never_____
2. When a youth asks a question which seems trivial or unimportant to me, I ignore him or jokingly scoff at his question.

3. I poke fun at, mock, tease, or ridicule individual youngsters.
   A. Often_____ B. Sometimes_____
   C. Rarely or never_____

4. I get the group or individuals to do what they are supposed to do by threatening them or warning of what I will do to them if they disobey.
   A. Often_____ B. Sometimes_____
   C. Rarely or never_____

5. I discourage "conning" and manipulation by reminding various youngsters that they can't con *me*, that I've got them pegged, can see right through them, know how their minds work, and what their game is.
   A. Often_____ B. Sometimes_____
   C. Rarely or never_____

6. Since many delinquents are not aware of how their bad personalities affect others, when I recognize a fellow's faults, I tell him what they are without his asking.
   A. Often_____ B. Sometimes_____
   C. Rarely or never_____

7. I figure out the real causes behind youngsters' delinquent behavior or personality problems, and explain to them how they got that way.
   A. Often_____ B. Sometimes_____
   C. Rarely or never_____

8. When one of the delinquent youths in my group says something insolent or defiant, especially in front of others, I take quick, direct, forceful action to prove who is boss.
   A. Often_____ B. Sometimes_____
   C. Rarely or never_____

9. Because delinquents need to learn social conformity, I make up rules and issue orders which have no real purpose in the program except training these young mavericks to follow rules and obey orders.
   A. Often_____ B. Sometimes_____
   C. Rarely or never_____

10. I criticize, reprimand, or chew out individuals in front of others.
    A. Often_____ B. Sometimes_____
    C. Rarely or never_____

11. I assign special responsibilities or privileges on the basis of which youngster are my favorites – the ones I like best.
    A. Often_____ B. Sometimes_____
    C. Rarely or never_____

12. I privately warn some members of the group not to associate with certain others who may be a bad influence on them.
    A. Often_____ B. Sometimes_____
    C. Rarely or never_____

13. When no program activities are scheduled and my group has time on its hands, in order to keep them from becoming bored, restless and troublesome, the best thing to do as group leader is to think of some activity and make them do it.
    A. Often_____ B. Sometimes_____
    C. Rarely or never_____

14. I assure these youths they may tell me all their problems, plans, thoughts and feelings – in strict confidence, and that this information will be kept confidential, and never used against them in any way.
    A. Often_____ B. Sometimes_____
    C. Rarely or never_____

15. I gain acceptance from my group of young delinquents by "speaking their language" – learning their slang, and using such terms as "punk," "fink" and "pig" in our everyday conversations.
    A. Often_____ B. Sometimes_____
    C. Rarely or never_____

16. When one of my group comes to me with a personal problem or complaint, I tell him where he is wrong, what he should do, and where his shortcomings lie.
    A. Often_____ B. Sometimes_____
    C. Rarely or never_____

17. I maintain control over my group, and prevent rebellion, by picking out the strongest, toughest individuals and giving them special status and privileges as my "assistants."
    A. Often_____ B. Sometimes_____
    C. Rarely or never_____

18. My group causes no trouble whenever I am on duty. They are loyal to me personally and won't put me in a bad light with my supervisors because they consider me "one of the boys." I gain this kind of loyalty and control through agreeing with the guys' delinquent values when no other authority figures are present.
    A. Often_____ B. Sometimes_____
    C. Rarely or never_____
19. I am changeable and unpredictable as to how I react to the youngsters' behavior, depending on what kind of mood I'm in at a given time.
    A. Often_____ B. Sometimes_____
    C. Rarely or never_____
20. I am uncomfortable while in charge of this group of untrustworthy and dangerous young con-men, hoods, and muggers. I dread coming to work and spending eight hours with them.
    A. Often_____ B. Sometimes_____
    C. Rarely or never_____

Okay. That's it. Let's see how you did.

Scoring

For each item you checked (A), score 1 point.
For each item you checked (B), score 2 points.
For each item you checked (C), score 3 points.

Add up all your points for a total score.

What Might Your Score Mean?³

Now, don't get all shook up if my interpretation of your quiz score doesn't quite match your impression of yourself. There are several reasons why this could occur. One is, I don't know you. Another is, you don't know me and didn't understand what I meant in the quiz items. Yet another might be that you don't know yourself.

In a few minutes we will go through the quiz items one by one. I will explain the principle I had in mind, and why, on each one. You can compare this with your own ideas and frame of reference. For all I know, your interpretations and methods of handling these situations are better than mine. Also, remember that exceptional circumstances pop up from time to time which call for emergency actions not covered by the general rules.

At any rate, here is my interpretation. If it doesn't fit you as you see yourself, read on and find out why. If it does fit, wear it. But read on anyway, to find out whether you gave all those neat answers by accident, for the right (my) reasons, or for some reasons of your own even better than mine.

IF YOUR TOTAL SCORE IS	THEN
57-60	You are a fantastic leader.
46-56	You are (or could be) a solid effective leader with delinquent youth, helping them to broaden their self-concepts and become more effective in their interactions with the world.
31-45	As of now, you would probably be happier and more effective as a guard outside the fence than as a youth worker inside. Keep studying human relations principles, though, and maybe try a few new experiences* to limber up your own fearful, overcontrolling, or otherwise rigid approach to human relations, and you could grow into a growth-inspiring leader.
20-30	Society would be much better off if its delinquent youth** never came into contact with you. Have you considered some other line of work?

*Such as an encounter group or an assertiveness training class.
**Or any other youth, for that matter.

Why Did You Answer It That Way?[4]

These are the principles I had in mind in writing each of the quiz items. Feel free to disagree, or to think up better ones from your own viewpoint and past experience.

(1) Punishing group for misbehavior of individuals

Don't do it. Great damage may be done to the innocent, strengthening their convictions that adults and authority figures are arbitrary, unfair and always out to "mess over" them. Better the guilty should go free than to punish the innocent — especially the innocent who has been struggling to "do good."

Imagine the young man who, having stolen something everyday for five years, has now strengthened his self-control and value system to the point where he has avoided temptation for three consecutive months. He is well on the road to eliminating thievery from his lifestyle. Now, one of his neighbors commits a theft, and the angry adult in charge, not knowing who did it, announces, "All right you guys. Somebody in here stole my cigarettes out of the office last night. I don't know who did it, so you six guys with beds nearest the office will stay here and mop the floor while the rest go to the movie this evening. One of you six probably did it."

What do you suppose is running through our young, nearly-reformed thief's mind that evening as he slaves over a hot mop while most of his friends are enjoying the movie? My guess is, it's something like, "That dirty *!xx#* counselor! I didn't steal no lousy cigarettes. I ain't stole nothin' for three months. And what does it get me? Miss the movie, mop the floor, and get called a thief. All right. I'll show that *!!xx*! If he's gonna treat me like a thief, I might as well act like one. He doesn't know what a real thief is. I'll show that *!!xx*!"

Thanks to this "youth leader's" inept handling of the problem, our young man's months of progress may be wasted — down the drain.

There are certain circumstances, however, under which a group may be held responsible for the behavior of its individual members. In fact, if used correctly, this method can be an effective means of inducing personality growth in individuals who lack a sense of identity at the level of responsible community membership. Peer group pressure can be harnessed to ride herd on these social mavericks until they begin to see themselves in a brand new light — as someone who "belongs" to the group, receives the wrath of the group for irresponsible behavior, and receives acceptance, recognition, and other forms of love as rewards for cooperative, civilized behavior.

"What's the difference," you ask, "between holding the group responsible for the behavior of its members and punishing groups for the misdeeds of individuals?" Okay, the difference is simple, but vital. In the deliberate, positive use of peer pressure to induce individual growth, the group must be advised *in advance* as to what its responsibilities are regarding the behavior of its individual members. They must be told what consequences, positive or negative, will befall the entire group as a result of individuals' actions. For example, "Gentlemen, ash trays have been provided. Cigarette butts on the floor are damaging to the carpet and a nuisance to clean up. In order for this group to retain dayroom smoking privileges, *everyone* is expected to do his part. *Any* cigarette butts found on the floor will result in immediate cancelation of this privilege for the whole group, and *all* smoking will have to be confined to the courtyard outside."

See the difference?

(2) Ignoring or scoffing at "trivial" questions

Who are you to judge that a question is unimportant *to the person who is asking it*? His concern may seem silly to you, with your greater knowledge and social sophistication, but it may be extremely serious and important to the troubled, naive youngster asking you for a helping hand in his struggle toward social adjustment and maturity.

Remember that many of these fouled-up kids see themselves as basically unloveable and unworthy of respect. The way to help is to *give* them acceptance and respect consistently until they are forced to change their own views of themselves. The new "self" which gradually emerges, feeling secure and worthy of acceptance as a human being, can then abandon its habitual defensiveness and delinquent attempts to "get even" with a rejecting world. One of the many simple, everyday methods of giving respect — treating with dignity — is to pay courteous attention to inquiries, and to answer them in a civil way.

Certainly there will be times when you are too busy supervising an activity or handling a crisis to take time right then to discuss some unrelated issue. But you can always take time to say, "I'm sorry, but you can see I'm really tied up right now. Let's discuss it later when there is more time."* It doesn't take any longer to say this than it does to tell him to shut up and quit annoying you with his stupid questions.

(3) Teasing, poking fun at, ridiculing, individuals

Teasing or poking fun is usually a thinly veiled form of cruelty. It is certainly not the prescribed medicine for young persons whose problems are rooted in feelings of inferiority and "unloveableness." They can do without further reminders of their inadequacies.

A surefire, never-fail method to destroy any spark of ambition toward self-growth a young man may have is to tease him by calling attention to his past shortcomings in the area in which he is trying to improve (e.g., "Well, miracles never cease. Look who's working! Old lazy butt himself. The world must be coming to an end.")

Ridicule is the poison. A sincere compliment is the medicine.

(4) Ruling by threat

You may be able to control a group of rebellious youths by constantly threatening them, especially if they are convinced that you have the power to carry out your threats.** You, brandishing the authority of your position, may hold an axe over their heads and receive compliance. But if you do — if this is your approach to youth leadership — you will fail utterly to inspire positive internal changes in their personalities. You will be frustrating their emotional needs, rather than satisfying them, and, consequently, you will be rejected as an ego model. The youths in your care will dislike you because you act as if you dislike them. And, as soon as you are no longer riding herd on them — when you are no longer in a position to carry

---

*But mean it! For cryin' out loud, don't use this as an excuse to put the youngster off, and then fail to talk with him about his question later.

**But woe unto you, brother, if you're bluffing and they call your hand.

out your threats — they will quit doing what you have been trying to "train" them to do, and probably do the exact opposite just for the hell of it.

There is a difference, sometimes hard to see, but vast, between personal threat and the impersonal clarification of reality — pointing out the consequences to be expected for certain behavior. Recognition of this difference is a quality which differentiates a correctional youth worker from an insecure, bullying tyrant. It is proper, and necessary, for the youth worker (and for parents) to explain the ground rules to their charges, to point out the realistic consequences of violations, and to *enforce* these consequences impartially and impersonally. Mostly through the *way* he says it, the good youth worker (and good parent) will get across the message that he sees the youths as responsible persons. Since he cares about them and wants them to avoid stumbling into trouble unintentionally, he wants to be sure they understand what is expected of them.

Incompetent Youth Worker: "All right, you guys. There's been talking after lights out and I know who is doing it. Now keep your mouths shut. Anyone makes a peep will answer to me personally. I'm gonna call security and have your butt tossed into lock-up for the night." (Here we have a man getting himself rejected as an ego model.)

Competent Youth Worker: "Okay, listen up a minute. Some of you have to get up at four-thirty to work the early shift in the kitchen, and I understand you've been having trouble getting to sleep because of talk after lights out. How about the rest of you showing your consideration? After all, we don't want these fellows to fall asleep and drown in the pancake batter." Here we see a good ego-model in action. He is accepted as an ego model because he is meeting the needs of the early shift by showing concern for their sleep problems; he is meeting the needs of the others by addressing them with dignity, as if he expects them to *want* to do the right thing. And what kind of characteristics is he displaying to those youths who are identifying with him? Warmth; human sensitivity and concern; courtesy; assumption of responsibility; use of authority without obnoxiously calling attention to it; and, not the least of these virtues, a sense of humor. These are exactly the kinds of ingredients the delinquent youths need to fill the empty spaces in their own impoverished personalities.

(5) Avoiding being "conned" by reminding the youths that you've got them pegged, can see right through them, are onto their game, etc.

A sense of personal integrity — a real feeling of "self" as a unique, worthwhile individual — is an essential part of emotional health. The youth worker should be aiming at *increasing* this sense of integrity — of wholeness — in his young charges. You are working in the opposite, or damaging, direction if you boast to a youth, or imply mysteriously, that you have him all figured out, as if he were an inanimate chemical compound under your microscope.

The delinquent youth is *not* a research project. He is a *person* who needs help, and you are a *person* trying to help him to mature and clarify his thinking, attitudes and feelings so that he can more effectively cope with life. You are trying to *help* him, not outsmart him or defeat him in some kind of contest. Subjecting him to detective games and staring at him through a microscope are not ways to help.

(6) Telling youngsters what their faults are when they haven't asked

Avoid telling a youth what his personal faults are when he has not asked your opinion. Often, even if he has asked you, criticism is not what he really wants to hear, and it is *not* what will help him. If your unsolicited criticism should be true, he will not believe you. He will defend himself, and will see you as an enemy (not an ego model), attacking and insulting him. If you are wrong in your diagnosis of his problems, you may cause him to waste a lot of energy going up the wrong alley.

Often when a youngster, especially one who is overly dependent, asks for your opinion of himself or something he did, he is trying to maneuver *you* into assuming responsibility for his decisions and behavior, and their improvement.* The wise youth leader will not fall for this. Don't accept this responsibility, for you can not follow

---

*He wants to use your ego instead of growing and exercising one of his own. It's easier that way.

this youngster through life to fulfill it. Encourage him to use his own developing ego. It needs the exercise. Shift the question and the responsibility back to him by asking, "How do you see yourself in that situation? What do you think of what you did?"

(7) Explaining to youths the "real causes" of their problems

Attempting to interpret personality dynamics (historical and unconscious factors which caused the present problems, or symptoms, to develop) is best left to professional clincians trained in the analytic psychotherapies.[5] A therapist telling a young man, for instance, that his burglaries represented a symbolic attempt to get love from his rejecting mother, might be appropriate in certain cases *after* having worked through his memories and painful feelings for many weeks, to the point where the young man is on the verge of gaining this "insight" himself, but can't quite put it together. At this point the therapist helps the youth to "crystalize" the formula he is trying to put together by advancing the "interpretation."

If you, as a day-by-day youth worker (or even if you are a professional clinician, for that matter), spring this fancy interpretation on our young burglar out of a clear blue sky, he may either ignore you as some kind of nut; be deeply hurt and develop a lot of anxiety or depression; or become very angry toward you for attacking his mother who, he likes to believe, certainly *does* love him.

(8) Proving who is boss by quick, forceful action against youths who speak defiantly

If you accept the challenge (for that's what it often is) when a youth in your care speaks defiantly or rudely, then two people instead of one will have to try to save face. Usually, you will win the contest by verbally "putting him in his place" in front of the group; by employing your greater physical strength (if you have it) or by physically putting him in his place by calling security staff to lock him up.[6] Yes, you can win the face saving contest, but you will probably be damaging the youth, not helping him. Embarrassment, shame, and inglorious defeat are not great ego builders.

Calmly recognizing a youth's angry feelings—looking at them as a symptom of a problem, rather than as a personal attack upon your honor — will permit you to handle the situation constructively. "Hey, you seem pretty mad at me. What's the problem?" This simple act of showing that you recognize that the youth *feels* angry, without counterattacking him, will usually cause him to simmer down, and he will start to tell you what's bugging him. Then you can meet his needs by helping him solve whatever the problem is, and he, consequently, will identify with you as an ego model and learn that there are better approaches to resolving conflicts than both sides blazing away with raw aggression.

An immature person with insecurity problems of his own (who shouldn't be a correctional youth worker in the first place) cannot do what needs to be done in situations like this. He is either compelled to vigorously defend his authority or, if insecure enough, to yield control of the situation to the angry, defiant youth, abdicating his role as leader.

A mature* youth worker with *true* authority knows he has it, and does not have to "prove it" to youths who express anger or defiance. He does not have to become defensive, and compete with delinquent youths on their own terms to show them who is "boss."

(9) Making up rules and orders which have no purpose except to train rebellious youth in obeying rules and orders

In the United States of America, the correctional youth worker should be helping his young clients to prepare for full membership in a democratic society. A democracy (at least the kind that Thomas Jefferson envisioned) operates under the premise that its members ought to be rational thinking people, not robots. Rules or laws in such a democracy are made by, or with the approval of, these rational, thinking people. It is their intention that each such rule or law serve a practical purpose toward their own welfare. Why then, should you train your youthful offenders to obey nonsense rules or orders?

Would it not be more useful and meaningful to help them to learn and practice some of the principles and methods of democracy? Explain the purpose and social values behind rules which you im-

---

*I'm not talking about any specific age, but about emotional and social maturity.

pose. Guide your charges in the formulation of some of their own rules, so they may begin to understand how the laws of our society (which they have violated) come into being. Help them learn that rules are not necessarily arbitrary nonsense, but have real purpose.

Blind obedience is not the hallmark of a healthy citizen, but understanding and respecting the rights of others is.

(10) Reprimanding in public

When you reprimand or criticize a youth (or anyone, for that matter) in the presence of his peers, you are in fact challenging him to defend himself — another face saving situation. If he successfully defends himself, you lose face. If he cannot defend himself, *he* loses face, and will hate you for crushing and embarrassing him.

Intolerable behavior by an individual in a group setting can usually be toned down with a quiet word or two. If more elaborate criticism or explanation is necessary, it can more effectively be given in private at a later time.

(11) Assigning special responsibilities and privileges to "favorites"

Obviously, this is favoritism, but you do *no* favor to a youth when you give him a special privilege on an arbitrary basis. Each such privilege is resented by the others in your group. The "privileged" one will be made to pay in one way or another — perhaps by being socially snubbed and rejected; perhaps by being called a "brown nose;" perhaps by being thumped, toe-stomped or rat packed.

Awarding special jobs on the basis of objectively demonstrable merit, or through election of candidates by the youths themselves, are a couple of ways to avoid the harmful effects of favoritism.

(12) Warning youths not to associate with certain others in the group who might be a bad influence on them

In advising Youth A not to associate with Youth B, you may *or may not* be doing Youth A a favor. You certainly are *not* helping Youth B, whom you are making a social outcast by your own behavior. You are reinforcing his old problem of feeling (and being) unloved and rejected.

Now, a parent has a perfect right to advise his own children to stay away from certain rotten kids in the neighborhood (or even insist upon it), because the parent's primary responsibility is the welfare of his own children. He has no obligation to care for and properly raise somebody else's delinquent kid. Not so, with you as youth worker. You have an obligation to be a good ego model and provide growth-inducing interpersonal experiences *for the bad guy as well as the good guy* in your group.

Can you see why you may not even be doing Youth A a favor by advising him to avoid Youth B? In so doing, you are communicating to Youth A that you think he is a weak, helpless creature with no ability to decide for himself whether or not to absorb the "bad" kid's badness. You are telling Youth A, "You are irresponsible. If I don't play mother hen, you are so weak and stupid you will become like the bad guy."

If Youth B hears, which he will, that you are advising his friends to reject him, he will think of you as a nosey, malicious busybody who has no right to interfere with any of his few legitimate sources of interpersonal happiness. And he will be right.

Think a minute. What you really want as a youth worker is not the dissolution of friendships. You want the friendships to be wholesome and growth-inducing. If the "bad" can rub off, why can't the "good"? It is possible to develop a program which will emphasize and reward the positive aspects of Youth A's relationship with Youth B and curtail the occurrence and minimize the impact of the negative features.[7] Under skillful leadership, these two can have beneficial effects on each other.

(13) Filling unscheduled program time by thinking up activities and making the group participate in them

That's the easy way, deciding arbitrarily what your group will do. It's better than providing no program at all, but, the growth-inducing experiences you can give your youngsters—feeling self-worth, self-responsibility, belongingness, and that an adult values their opinions—are well worth the extra effort in permitting the group to participate in planning its own program.

(14) Guaranteeing confidentiality—privileged communication

Man, you can't do that! You can't guarantee to a delinquent youth that he may tell you anything—all his past activities and plans for the future—with absolute assurance that you will keep it under your hat. Well, you can tell him that if you want to, but only at the risk of being a liar or a criminal. What if he tells you "in confidence" that he is the one who committed those six unsolved murders in his neighborhood last year? Or that a buddy on "the outs" smuggled a gun to one of the guys in the dorm next door, and he plans to use it tonight to shoot the night supervisor and escape? In spots like these, you either have to back down on your guarantee of confidentiality or become an accessory to a crime.

One major purpose of a treatment program for delinquents is to replace false, stereotyped attitudes toward the adult world with fair, realistic ones. It is necessary to *demonstrate* in such a program that all adults are *not* unloving, uncaring, unfeeling and untrustworthy. Obviously, violating a youngster's confidence is not a good way to show him that adults can be trustworthy. And you most certainly are not being a model of concern for the lives and welfare of your fellowmen if you have knowledge of past or impending crimes and fail to take appropriate action to protect society.

How did you get into this mess? Why did you guarantee confidentiality in the first place? People are going to tell you only what they feel is safe, whether or not they have been given a promise of confidentiality. I have had youths voluntarily confess past crimes knowing full well they would be held accountable for them. I've also known people who held back information from their lawyers, therapists or priests when confidentiality *was* guaranteed because they were too ashamed to talk about it, or didn't trust the guarantee *that* much.

I don't believe that a guarantee of confidentiality, or the lack of one, has much influence on what, or how much, is said in a counseling setting. If you feel compelled to make an issue of it with your clients, or if they should come right out and ask if they can tell you something in strict confidence, I suggest something along these lines:

> I am interested in hearing anything you want to talk about. You may express any feelings you want to, or any problems, and I will try to be helpful. You should know, though, that I have a responsibility not only to help you if I can, but also for

the welfare of other people. If someone gives me some information that makes me believe that they, or someone else is in danger of being harmed in some way, then I will do whatever I feel is necessary to prevent the damage from being done. I won't promise to cover up crimes. That would make me guilty of them — an accomplice.

(15) "Speaking the language" of delinquents in order to gain their acceptance

I have no quarrel with the use of slang, per se, nor am I pushing for cold, formal, musty language as the "acceptable" means of communicating in a correctional program.

What concerns me is that many slang terms in the delinquents' vernacular reflect false, distorted, perceptions of reality. If you, as the adult ego model, use such terms in the same contexts — terms based on, and reflecting, the antisocial views and values which led these youths into trouble — you are unwittingly expressing agreement with the twisted values. If you, for example, refer disparagingly to someone as a "fink," you are telling your delinquent charges that you agree with THE CODE — that you share their screwed-up belief that anyone who reports a crime is a bad person — a "fink."

As a correctional youth worker, you are supposed to be helping these immature people to develop sound, rational, adult values. You are not supposed to be doing it the other way around — identifying with the delinquents' values and learning to behave like a cool dude or bad mutha.

(16) Telling youths with problems, what is "wrong" with them

Hold your tongue, knave! Often when a troubled youth approaches you with "a problem to talk over," he doesn't have a concrete problem at all, and he is not looking for criticism or advice. Instead, he is frightened, depressed or angry, not exactly sure why, and is in fact looking for a receptive listener he can trust. He needs someone who will listen *without* attacking or criticizing, who will understand how he feels, and who will let him unload his pent up painful feelings. *After* this has been done, some concrete problems may emerge, and it may become appropriate to help him clarify them and suggest some possible solutions.

Almost never does a disturbed youth approach the youth worker in the hope of hearing a lecture, being told how much better you did it when you were a boy, or what is wrong with him. Even if a dependent type youngster should ask for such structure, and mean it, you can probably best help him by refusing to let him become overly dependent upon you to do his thinking for him. Listen. Encourage him, and guide him when necessary, to think things through, look for and evaluate alternatives, and develop solutions for his own problems.

(17) (Maintaining control by appointing strong "assistants" from the group, giving them special status or privileges for their support

Maintaining control by placing one youth in a position of authority over other members of the group amounts to abdicating your responsibility as leader. Unfortunately, this is sometimes done formally by appointing "officers" or "monitors," and sometimes informally by subtly or secretly offering special status or good grades in return for the "helpful" cooperation of a "Have Muscles, Will Travel." Either way, it is bad news.

A pleasant interpersonal atmosphere where "control" is maintained through cooperation and mutual respect is achieved by supervising according to the principles of courtesy, fairness and personal integrity. Fearful obedience by delinquent youths can be achieved by appointing stronger peers who threaten them. Their *respect* has to be earned. But which do you think really gives you the most effective and secure "control"? Which is most likely to result in personality growth?

(18) Gaining loyalty and control by becoming "one of the boys"— by agreeing with delinquent values—when other adults are not present

"Personalizing" your control of a group by becoming "one of the boys" when alone with them, using their antisocial language in their contexts, applauding delinquent values, or boasting of your own illegal or immoral adventures, may be even more damaging to these young people than the opposite approach of rejecting, dominating, criticizing and moralizing. The holier-than-thou "leader," failing to meet the youth's emotional needs, is not accepted as an ego model and, therefore, has little or no effect on the youths, except for temporarily annoying them. You, however, through playing the friend, supporting their antisocial attitudes, and being a "regular" guy, may be meeting a number of the youngsters' needs, thus encouraging the identification process. Stop it! Man, they don't need to become like you. They are already that way. That is their problem.

If your group's good behavior is based on their thinking of you as a secret member of the gang, you are pulling a dirty trick on your co-workers on other shifts who do not believe in encouraging the youngsters in their antisocial attitudes and values. If this is your approach to earning a paycheck as a youth leader, you ought to be *in* a personality development program instead of supervising one.

(19) Being unpredictable in responding to youths' behavior, depending on mood

Principles of good leadership and healthful interpersonal relationships will serve much better than moods and emotional impulses in guiding your behavior toward the youngsters in your care.

To counteract the poison produced by a youth's unpredictable, unreliable, cold, unfriendly early relationships with adults, the antidote is consistent, reliable, warm, friendly relationships over a period of time with other adults.

It is impossible for youngsters to absorb stable, consistent values and social response patterns from an adult model who acts friendly one day and unfriendly the next, or who interprets rules, restrictions, program and discipline differently, depending on whether he got a raise, had a flat tire on the way to work, or had a spat with his spouse at breakfast.

I'm not suggesting that the youth leader should be a cold fish. Happiness, sadness and anger are normal human emotions. They do not need to be kept under lock and key. They should not, however, be allowed to dominate the youth leader's rational self to the point where his reactions to the youths in his care become inconsistent, unpredictable and confusing to them.

(20) Dreading to come to work

If, over the months, you frequently dread "putting up with" the group of youths with whom you work, you cannot be fully effective as a youth leader.

There are any number of possible causes for such feelings. It could be that you are simply in the wrong line of work. Some people work most comfortably with other people; some with mechanical equipment; some with musical instruments; some with papers, pencils and typewriter; some with their muscles; and some with their mouths.* Perhaps your best field is not people — or especially, delinquent people.

Another possibility is that you have unwittingly adopted a competitive, instead of helping attitude toward your charges. Perhaps you think of your work with them as a kind of daily contest. They are constantly striving to put something over on you or "get their own way," while you are striving to keep ahead of them and prevent them from outsmarting you. This can become exhausting.

It is also possible that most of your discomfort is coming from some other areas of your life (marital, financial, etc.), and that your group of difficult delinquent youngsters just adds one more straw to the proverbial camel's back.

The point is that, *whatever* the cause may be, if your feelings toward the youths in your care, and your interactions with them, are negative, uncomfortable, angry, fearful, grouchy, suspicious, or punitive, then the interpersonal relationships which you can offer them will not inspire the growth process we hope for. You will not be able to provide the antidote for the negative relationships that retarded their social and emotional growth in earlier years.

Should the preceding paragraph apply to you as a youth worker, you have several options. You may ignore your problem and continue to perform your job unhappily and incompetently. You might explore some personal vocational counseling to determine if you have stumbled into a field which is incompatible with your interests and aptitudes. Or, *personality* counseling could reveal emotional conflicts which are making you incompatible with the requirements

---

*Hopefully in cooperation with their brains.

of your job as a youth worker. A bonus is that this last option can do more than identify your conflicts. It can also resolve them, enabling you to work comfortably and effectively with youth.

NOTES

1. The effects of delinquent youths upon each other can be terrible to excellent, depending upon whether the adult leaders are really leading, and have structured a program to encourage and reward positive behavior.

2. If you don't feel like messing up this book with a bunch of check marks, grab a piece of scratch paper and number from 1 to 20. After the number of each item place the letter designating your answer—A, B, or C.

3. This is not supposed to be a standardized test. So, for any psychologist looking in let's not waste time quibbling about validity and reliability. The purposes of the quiz are to stimulate some "Who am I?"-type thinking in the reader regarding his abilities, or potential abilities, as a people worker, and to open the door to discussion of the human relations principles behind the questions.

4. This quiz may be used as a training device with groups of correctional workers. In a group setting, discussion of the individual items can be rich and rewarding as the participants share their personal viewpoints and experiences, and add them to those of the writer.

5. Later in the chapter on "Withdrawn Willie Comes Alive," we will see how professional analytic therapy can make a delinquent get worse instead of better, and also how, used with the right person, at the right time, *and in conjunction with the right other techniques*, analytic therapy can help clear up problems often considered "untreatable."

6. Of course, on rare occasions it may become necessary to control a situation quickly and forcefully to prevent it from erupting into bedlam, but such crises occur much less frequently than some youth workers seem to believe. Most often they could have been prevented by using skillful, nondefensive tactics in the first place.

7. More about program development coming up, next chapter.

Chapter VII

Escalon:
Birth of an Upstart Program

What happens if you train some youth workers in the leadership style and human relations philosophy discussed in the previous chapter, add some formal individual and group treatment methods, and turn these features into a specialized program for the most severely maladjusted and disruptive youths in a traditional correctional institution? In this chapter we will take a backward look at just such a pioneer program.

BACKGROUND

In October, 1956 I accepted a position with the State of California, Department of the Youth Authority. In those days, each Youth Authority institution was entitled to one psychologist, no matter how many hundreds of court-committed delinquent youths were housed therein. My remote outpost was the Paso Robles School for Boys, about halfway between Los Angeles and San Francisco. My clients were 350 young men between ages 14 and 18 (soon expanded to 450) committed to the State of California for offenses ranging from possession of a can of beer[1] to murder.

Upon my arrival, the school, a compound of low, Spanish style, red brick buildings, ringed by golden barley fields and oak-studded hillocks, sprawled lazily in the shimmering October heat. The then modern 1956 facilities of the institution—a self-contained mini-state with its own farm, kitchen, bakery, laundry, shoe repair shop, academic school, and library—were a far cry from what had been there in 1947 when it was opened on a 200-acre piece property acquired from the United States Government. Its first dormitories, classrooms, shops and offices had been converted from wooden barracks abandoned by the old Estrella Army Air Corps Base. It was drafty (Paso Robles winter nights frequently drop to eighteen degrees), non-fireproof, heated by old oil stoves, and plagued by erratic plumbing of uncertain vintage. Some of the original buildings had burned down mysteriously in the middle of the night, according to "old timers" who had been recruited from neighboring farms as the institution's first youth workers.

These staff, who had undergone hardships together, shared many rich experiences, and handled many gut-level crises, all without help from some ivy-covered scholar, were not wildly enthusiastic about my potential for improving "their" programs. A couple of other psychologists had preceded me in the position, and had been accepted by staff, largely, from what I heard, because they were nice fellows who mostly stayed in their offices and had individual youths come in for testing, counseling, or "whatever psychologists do with them."

I was not in a position to carry on the tradition of my predecessors. At that time, the Youth Authority statewide, had begun to suspect that the traditional human warehouse-type institutions were not effective at improving attitudes, values and behavior. The Superintendent of the Paso Robles School, Gerald Spencer, knew that "treatment" was in the wind. He was aware that the Youth Authority knew very little about correctional treatment. Whatever it was, if it would help troubled kids, he wanted it in his programs. Consequently, when I took the job at Paso Robles, it was with the explicit understanding that I would *not* just stay in my office and do whatever it is that psychologists do. I agreed to do everything in my power to integrate real treatment concepts and methods into the Paso Robles correctional program (with no money in the budget for that purpose). Mr. Spencer wanted his institution to become a "treatment facility," whatever that was, and hired me to try to bring it about. If he had *not* wanted it, and had not supported my efforts administratively at critical times, I would have been ridden out of town on a rail.

The plan was for me to ease into the situation — to absorb a full two weeks of orientation and get fully acquainted with staff and existing program before taking on any clinical work. Plans go astray.

My second day on the job, in an orientation meeting with the superintendent and some other administrative staff, the door burst open and a wrought up security man bellowed, "We got back that crazy Cromwell* kid! He's out of his head. We've got him locked in a security room, but he's raising hell. Screaming and trying to kick the walls down. Where's that new psychologist?"

"Who is the Cromwell kid?" I asked Superintendent Spencer.

"Well, he's mostly been trouble for us. Been here about four months, and nobody has been able to do a thing with him. Fights staff like a tiger rather than go back to the cottage he is assigned to. Won't say why. He's been in segregation for the past two weeks, and day before yesterday he escaped. I guess they just got him back."

"Maybe I'd better have a look?"

"Yes, I think you'd better."

Thus ended what was perhaps the only two-week orientation ever completed in two days. Young Harry Cromwell became my first clinical client in the Youth Authority, and, perhaps more important in the overall scheme of things, he became the first I identified of a group of extremely disturbed, maladaptive youngsters whose personalities were so unsuited to the traditional institutional routine that they were being terribly damaged by it. They—ten of them, referred rapidly from all living units as soon as word got around to staff that I had taken Harry Cromwell off of someone's hands— became the original population of Escalon, the Youth Authority's pioneer treatment program.

I suppose, before discussing the treatment program itself, you would like to hear the rest about Harry Cromwell—why he was raising so much hell and running away, and what we were able to do about it. Maybe I should tell you but I won't, because this chap-

---

*All names of the delinquent youths in this book have been changed.

ter is about the treatment program, not Harry Cromwell. But don't worry about Heinous Harry. He has Chapter X all to himself.*

ESCALON—A STEP
TOWARD REAL CORRECTIONS

This program was undertaken in advance of an anticipated Youth Authority-wide movement toward more effective correctional treatment for two reasons. First, wards (the term used to designate youths committed to the Youth Authority) with severe personality problems were already present. They needed whatever treatment could be mustered without waiting for the resources eventually to be provided by the slow-turning, rusty wheels of bureaucracy. Second, it was hoped that Escalon[2] would clear a path for larger scale treatment programs to come. Many conflicts are generated when treatment philosophy and methods are suddenly superimposed upon traditionally custody-and-control-oriented institutions.[3]

Escalon attempted to integrate formal individual and group therapy with a therapeutic *milieu* — a total environment planned to provide informal growth-inducing interpersonal experiences throughout the day. Such a total push approach is the only way to go. Through the years, psychotherapy, individual and group, has bogged down whenever the everyday living program developed snags (e.g., acquiring a new youth worker who nagged, threatened, humiliated, or in other ways failed to treat the wards with respect), and has resumed progress when the environmental problem was corrected. It seems that people lose interest in exploring their inner selves when their outer selves are being mistreated.

The ten wards in Escalon were housed in one wing of the Potrero (discipline unit) building, not because that was the best place to put the program, but because it was the *only* place available. Each ward had his own room, decorated according to his individual tastes. The rooms, containing books and hobby craft, were cheerful and attractive — a far cry from the stark, death-cell green dorms and cubicles

---

*Of course, if you're the sneaky type, somewhat lacking in ego strength, you could furtively thumb ahead and read it now out of context. If you do, though, don't forget to come back.

which prevailed throughout the rest of the institution.* Except for being fairly neat and orderly, inspired by intragroup competition, the Escalon rooms closely resembled the bedrooms of teenage boys in an average home.[4]

A fifteen-foot chain link fence surrounding the living unit, courtyard and sports area was primarily for the benefit of transient discipline cases sharing the same building. The Escalon wards, enthused about their program and participating in its ongoing planning, showed practically no inclination to escape. Their activities were not confined to the unit. They often could be found, with their supervisor, in diverse areas of the campus, planting gardens, flying the model airplanes they had built, playing baseball, or enjoying some other imaginative activity the group had elected to pursue.

Morning program was supervised by a staff teacher who was also certified as a school psychologist. This educational phase of the program was aimed first at providing a wholesome interpersonal environment in which the wards could consistently experience feelings of self-respect, "group belongingness," and being a valued person in the eyes of an adult. The secondary aim was to neutralize the negative feelings most of the wards shared toward school. To overcome the affects of past failures and embarrassments in the classroom, each youngster was encouraged to select, in consultation with the teacher, the subjects he wanted to work on. Assignments and teacher assistance were then individualized according to interests and achievement levels. There was no inter-student competition, and individual accomplishments were consistently rewarded with public praise.

This need-oriented, noncoercive approach to teaching, often supplemented by the psychotherapeutic removal of emotional blocks to learning, enabled a number of young men with histories of miserable academic adjustment to enjoy school for the first time in their lives, and to achieve significant scholastic gains.

From noon until bedtime the program was guided by a carefully selected and trained group supervisor. Since this person was to serve as an ego model—a symbolic and corrective substitute for parents whose relationships with their children had frequently been

---

*We painted them *all* prettier colors a couple of years later.

pathological—it was essential that he be a stable and sensitive person who could grasp the concepts of therapeutic human relationships, and whose own personality was compatible with carrying them out. In selecting this supervisor and his successors in the program, personal characteristics sought included flexible thinking (the ability to look at a situation from several different perspectives); sensitivity to the feelings of others; sufficient freedom from personal insecurity to permit rational, nondefensive handling of hot emotional outbursts; a genuine liking for people; the ability to maintain rapport; warmth; firm moral convictions; and the ability to perceive, confront, and thwart attempted manipulations and deceptions by his charges.[5]

Afternoon and evening program was keynoted by flexibility. Activities, as much as possible, were determined democratically by the group itself.

I held a formal "brainstorming" session with the Escalon wards, in which they were instructed to spew out for a ten minute period, as many ideas for enriching and broadening their program as they could think of. They were asked to be creative, uninhibited and not to hold anything back because it might seem farfetched or silly. For now, we wanted creativity; screening the ideas for feasibility was a later step in the process. I told them that I would take all their ideas to the superintendent afterward, to see which of them he would approve for use in the program.

These "dull," "disturbed," "incompetent," "unimaginative" youngsters presented me with one hundred and forty-four suggestions in ten minutes flat. As promised, I took the list to the superintendent. He approved fifty-eight of the items as administratively feasible.[6] I reported back to Escalon with the approved list, and we began to plan the implementation of these activities. All fifty-eight ideas were eventually put into action—some of them revolutionary in the sense that they had never been done in the history of the institution. As a product of this experience, the "Escalonians" were able to see firsthand that "the establishment" is not always against them, and that legitimate channels exist through which they can have a voice in their own welfare.

A few of the new activities which emerged from the young brainstormers' heads and became program realities were a zoo (stocked initially with a wild rabbit pursued on foot and caught by one of the wards, and two pigeons donated by the Potrero unit's senior group supervisor); planting and raising vegetables and melons in individual gardens (with subsequent cookouts to make good use of the crops); music instruction; art; television viewing (a portable set was donated by one of the ward's parents); attending movies downtown (through the courtesy of the local theater manager); bowling instruction (volunteered by a nearby alley manager); boxing lessons; and monthly outings such as fishing trips and beach parties.[7]

Wards, deemed in need of it by the psychologist, were offered individual therapy as needed, as well as group therapy twice a week. Participation in the therapy group was voluntary. Usually six to eight attended while the remainder preferred to continue working with hobbycraft, read or engage in some other less anxiety-provoking pursuit. Group therapy was kept voluntary for two main reasons. One was that the participants needed the dignity afforded by choice — being able to make decisions about their own treatment. The other was that some individuals, due to shaky personality structures, intense anxiety, or low interpersonal maturity level, could not tolerate the small group process, or couldn't understand what it was all about and felt lost and rejected in the group. Many of these non-groupers, after a few months in the program, including an appropriate form of individual therapy, became strong enough to handle the group interaction, and began attending.

At the end of its first year, Escalon had survived many difficulties, the foremost of which was bitter resistance and repeated sabotage by a faction of hostile, "pure custody-oriented staff" who were confused and threatened by the relaxed, friendly, courteous relationships among Escalon staff and wards. They seemed to fear the possibility of being asked by "administration" to behave similarly towards their own wards (whom they had generally been able to control thus far through traditional authoritarian suppressive methods). This philosophical and methodological conflict was intensified by the unfortunate location of Escalon in the same building, sharing facilities (and sometimes even staff coverage), with the punishment-oriented disciplinary Potrero program. One Potrero program staff member complained about the conflict he experienced when he had to provide Escalon coverage, "I turn the corner and I'm supposed to quit scowling and smile. Then, when I come back I have to scowl again. Hell, I get mixed up and smile at the wrong guys.'' Survival of the program was made possible by ongoing communications provided by weekly staff meetings. Issues were brought out, fought out, and resolved.

Another problem was group composition. We learned the hard way that certain types of individuals didn't fit this type of program. For example, full-blown psychotics, ranting and raving, couldn't participate meaningfully, and spoiled the program for the others. (Several borderline psychotic wards, however, stabilized and did very well in Escalon.) A few moderately mentally retarded wards didn't seem to harm the program, but gained little, if anything, from it. Aggressive, power-striving sociopaths were incapable of real group interaction. They attempted to use the program as an arena for seeking prestige and status, becoming destructive, overbearing and disruptive. Flamboyant homosexuals generated anxiety among many wards with psychosexual identification problems. They sometimes stimulated their peers' latent homosexual trends into consciousness and overt expression. More often, they precipitated a deluge of neurotic anxiety and other symptoms against these taboo impulses.

Despite these difficulties, or perhaps *because* of them and the experience gained in overcoming them, at the end of that first year, I had some suggestions for the Youth Authority in its anticipation of developing ''official'' special treatment programs. These suggestions[8] included:

A. Clear channel two-way communications, vertically among treatment staff, and horizontally between treatment staff and regular training program personnel, are essential to the avoidance of confusion, suspicion, and resistance. Clarifying publications, frequent staff conferences, and in-service training meetings devoted to exchange of information among various services within the institution are effective means of minimizing frictions and misunderstanding.

B. Treatment staff must *experience* democratic leadership and constructive group interaction if they are to pass the effects of these therapeutic processes down to the patients.[9] Leaders lead, as a rule, not in a way they are instructed to lead, but in the way that *they are led*. It is nearly impossible for a supervisor to carry out a democratic, permissive[10] program with wards if he is subjected to an autocratic, dictatorial form of leadership himself.

C. An adequate in-service training program for treatment staff is essential. Personnel, especially those drawn from regular correctional programs, will have to be taught the concepts and methods of therapy.

D. Selection of staff who will exercise supervisory status over patients must be done carefully in order to eliminate persons whose own personal adjustment problems would foster destructive, rather than corrective, relationships with the patients.

E. Selection of patients for treatment groups must be based on professional knowledge of personality and group dynamics . . . Otherwise, poorly balanced groups and inappropriate individual cases can counteract all therapeutic efforts.

F. If treatment is going to involve more than psychotherapy, namely, the at least equally valuable benefits of small group interaction, the usual 50-ward cottages must house several subgroups with separate daily programs aimed at maintaining the unity of the corrective family-substitute groupings. Similarly, staff must be employed in a manner which will maximize each subgroup's time with the same leader, rather than allowing individuals to drift in a 50-ward crowd, and the shifting of "father figures"[11] so rapidly that no corrective family-substitute experiences can develop.

G. (At least) two different kinds of special treatment programs are needed. One is for types of patients whose maladjustments are amenable to treatment in a permissive, small group program. The other is for the less treatable group whose sociopathic, aggressive, or sexual disturbances would disrupt a permissive program, and whose needs demand a long-term, highly structured, and secure program as protection against their own impulses. Although both programs could be managed under the same administration, they would almost certainly have to be housed in separate buildings, and would

involve quite different modes of operation. Attempts to meet
the opposed needs of these two broad categories of wards in a
single living unit and program . . . can lead only to chaos and
failure to achieve effective treatment of either group.

The above observations have been heeded by the developers of
the many special purpose treatment programs now in operation
across the state. Many headaches have thereby been avoided or
eliminated.

The Escalon program, the alien infant, as it grew up over the next
three years, had some interesting effects on the rest of the institution. Some of these were direct outgrowths of Escalon. Others
sprang up in relatively remote soil, but unmistakably were products
of the high-morale atmosphere radiated by Escalon staff and wards.

Four new specialized programs, spinoffs from Escalon, were (1)
the Nipomo treatment program, (2) the Potrero treatment program,
(3) diagnostic staff conferences, and (4) the group counseling program.

THE NIPOMO TREATMENT PROGRAM

A warm, democratically-oriented, small group living program as
an approach to treating disturbed delinquent youths is superior to an
impersonal, cold, autocratic, regimented, mass living regime. At
Paso Robles, Escalon provided the preferred milieu, but for only
ten boys. Many others needed such a program. To accomplish this,
the Nipomo treatment program was initiated in May, 1958.

The Escalon group was increased from ten to fourteen and moved
from quarters in the discipline unit to Nipomo, a newly built fifty-
bed cottage. The cottage was then filled by adding thirty-six additional youths who were referred by line staff, interviewed by the
psychologist and identified as suffering social and emotional maladjustments which might respond favorably to a therapeutic commu-
nity-type program. These thirty-six were then divided into two
groups of eighteen, each with its own identity and separate daily
program.

Thus, Nipomo cottage came to house three small living groups,
rather than one large one. The three sections were together only for

the pre-bedtime evening period and for breakfast, lunch and dinner in the institution's main dining room.

Escalon continued to function independently, having its academic program in the cottage each morning, and a relatively unstructured, democratically chosen program of activities in the afternoons.

The academic programs of Nipomo A and Nipomo B were patterned after Escalon's. The structures of the "corrective family substitute groupings" were maintained by assigning each section, *as a group*, to one teacher, rather than scattering them among the population according to achievement test scores, the standard procedure. Academic achievement was considered secondary to the goal of improving social and emotional adjustment through experiencing positive interpersonal relationships and democratic leadership. Nipomo teachers were trained and functionally supervised by the institution's psychologist regarding their roles as counselor-teachers.[12]

The two Nipomo sections were charged with doing the laundry for the entire institution. Nipomo A worked the laundry in the mornings while B was in the classroom. In the afternoons these assignments were reversed.

Twice weekly, during class time, Escalon and each of the Nipomo sections were divided in half for group counseling. (All Escalon-Nipomo staff were trained in this skill.) Each teacher kept half of his class. The other half accompanied a designated group supervisor to another room for their small group session.

The Nipomo program also included recreation time, sports, religious opportunity and occasional off-campus outings.

The Escalon-Nipomo operation demonstrated how imaginative programming can overcome many budgetary and architectural limitations in establishing the small group environment vital to effective treatment, at least for a portion of the residents.

THE POTRERO TREATMENT PROGRAM

During the implementation of Escalon it became apparent that certain types of personalities could not profit from a permissive, democratically-oriented program. Further, they tended to destroy such an atmosphere. Those whose uncontrolled behavior, sociopathic, aggressive or sexual, disrupted a program such as Escalon, needed a treatment program of a different kind. These individuals required a long-term, highly structured and secure program that would contain their destructive behavior and protect them from their own impulses. The Potrero treatment program was designed for this purpose.

Potrero cottage was the institution's lock-up unit for transient disciplinary cases. After Escalon moved out to the new Nipomo cottage, Potrero staff, already familiar with the concepts and methods of environmental therapy, decided to attempt the highly structured kind of program needed by incorrigible, impulse-ridden, sociopathic or psychotic[13] wards.

The five or six residents of this program were wards whose disruptive behavior prohibited an acceptable adjustment anywhere else. Often they were boys who, while assigned to regular cottages, spent about half of their time in lock up for repeated infractions. The thought was, "Why not just keep them there, instead of shuffling them back and forth, and plan a special program for them?"

In essence, the program consisted of a highly structured set of activities, including calisthenics, manual work (e.g., chopping weeds), and academic school, interspersed with regularly scheduled individual and group counseling. Staff were selected and trained to provide an atmosphere of warm personal acceptance, and to be fair but firm in the exercise of their authority. Without great fanfare, acting out and manipulation simply were not permitted.

Residents could be paroled directly from the Potrero program, or when appropriate, they were transferred to a less structured program in transition to parole.

There are probably a few residents in every institution who, at least for a time, can be helped only by such a secure, highly structured, yet treatment-oriented program.

Potrero staff met weekly with the psychologist to discuss cases and the program. They were justifiably proud of their successful efforts to rehabilitate some of the most severely disturbed and unmanageable members of the institution's population.

DIAGNOSTIC CONFERENCES

Personal appearance staffing conferences, long used in mental hospitals for ongoing evaluation of patients' progress, were not used in Youth Authority facilities prior to their introduction in Escalon-Nipomo. Traditional classification reports had been submitted independently by each cottage staff member to the Classification Committee. The reports, concerned largely with the one behavioral variable, conformity, or obedience, were used by the committee as a basis for vital program decisions such as parole and transfers. The wards were seen by the committee only to inform them of what decision had been made.

The system introduced in Escalon-Nipomo featured a new written form which called for discussion of each ward's social interaction, values, moods, methods of handling frustration, sexual orientation, manner of thinking, and self-concept. These discussions, led by the cottage classification counselor, included all staff who worked with the ward — cottage personnel, teachers and tradespeople — and the ward himself. The psychologist acted as consultant on technical problems and cases with whose treatment he was directly involved.

The written summary of the staffing, highlighting each ward's personality, response to treatment, developmental trends, behavioral contract negotiations and results, provided the Classification Committee with really meaningful data upon which to base decisions.

Several advantages of the diagnostic staff conferences, beyond producing improved classification became evident. Staff intercommunications and morale improved. Cottage program became more consistent and productive as the improved communications produced greater consistency in staff values and goals. The age-old problem of wards accusing individual staff members of personal persecution was all but eliminated, as honest and open discussions involving all parties concerned replaced the old "secret ballot" classification reports.

Staff members from other cottages were invited to observe Escalon-Nipomo staffings and were offered assistance in developing their own. The psychologist followed up with staff meetings focused on the need to observe total personality adjustment, rather than just the subordination-insubordination factor. Other components of personality adjustment were identified and discussed. Each staff member was given a written guide sheet explaining this concept and describing illustrative kinds of behavior. Within a year, every cottage in the institution converted to the personal appearance diagnostic staff conference. Today it is prevalent in every institution and forestry camp in the Youth Authority.

THE GROUP COUNSELING PROGRAM

Due to early experiences with rejecting adults, many Youth Authority wards have come to think of all adults as cold, harsh, unloving taskmasters who preach and demand certain kinds of behavior without giving anything in return. Naturally, they will try to resist such preaching from persons they see as their natural enemies.

Group counseling permits a youth of this kind to straighten out his confused and antisocial feelings. He compares experiences with peers, receives personal acceptance, understanding, and respect from the other group members, and clears the hatred out of his system without fear of punishment or adult criticism.

Escalon-Nipomo wards were not the only ones in need of group counseling. A large-scale program covering the entire institution was needed. The problem was how to accomplish it.

Best results cannot be obtained if there are more than six to eight members in a group. It must meet consistently at least once a week if the intra-group relationships are to develop to the point where the members really trust each other and feel free to express themselves. If the goal is to provide such treatment for 450 boys, in groups of six, each group meeting once a week, 75 meetings must be held each week. One trained counselor would have to work 75 hours a week to accomplish this. Seventy-five trained counselors, each working one hour a week in this capacity, could accomplish it also. An approximation of the latter approach seemed the more practical of the two.

The next question was, "Where can we get 75 trained group counselors?" As it seemed unlikely that the state finance department would approve a request for 74 additional professional staff members, an expedient answer seemed to be, "Train any interested people who are already here to be group counselors."

Group counseling techniques are quite special and do not consist of "common sense," advice-giving, lecturing on morality, or being "buddy-buddy." In addition to reading about group counseling techniques, it is essential that the group counselor trainee observe them in operation or, better yet, experience them as a member of a counseling group. For this reason, several training groups were formed whose members were volunteer staff personnel interested in learning the process of group counseling.

This method of training was selected also because a group counselor, or any psychotherapist, can be effective only to the extent that his own personality is free of neurotic conflicts which interfere with his ability to allow clients to express themselves in all areas. Membership in a training group provides an opportunity for scanning oneself, gaining personal insights, recognizing one's own areas of neurotic adjustment, and correcting them.

Many of the staff members who participated in training groups, ". . . just to see what it is all about," without intending to conduct groups, reported that they derived satisfaction from the experience and found some of the concepts and techniques valuable in their everyday relationships, both business and social. Some of these people also wound up conducting ward groups.

Within a year more than forty staff members became volunteer members of counseling groups. Many of them, as they gained group process proficiency, started volunteer groups with wards. Trainees included all ten senior group supervisors, many group supervisors, six teachers, four classification counselors, four stenographers, one nurse, one school principal, one chaplain, one assistant head group supervisor, and the superintendent. These groups tended to average about twenty meetings in duration, although one was active over a year.

These staff were able to provide group counseling to the more than two hundred wards who requested it. These meetings were mostly scheduled for the hour immediately after regular bedtime. Since each group met only once per week, nobody was deprived of a significant amount of sleep.

DIFFUSE RADIATION EFFECT

In addition to the tangible program developments just described, many employees expressed the feeling that an unquantifiable change in the total atmosphere of the institution occurred gradually during the development of the Escalon program and its offspring, and that in some vague way the two sets of conditions were related. This diffuse radiation effect, if it is such, was usually discussed in terms of higher morale, friendlier everyday behavior among staff and wards alike, improved and more relaxed communications, more inspired work, far fewer gang fights and escapes, less tension, and less general turmoil.

A small treatment program, planted where the soil is fertile, and protected during its infancy, can mature, scatter seeds, and eventually dominate the institutional garden, just as a small patch of dichondra can spread in a lawn. The democratic leadership, warm human relations, mutual respect, and empathy which are the components of a treatment environment, if given a fair start, turn out to be basically stronger rewards than the display of cold authority in a regimented, impersonal, sheerly custodial program. That is what happened at Paso Robles.

NOTES

1. A few judges in remote counties which had little delinquency hardly ever got to commit anyone to the State, so naturally, they took advantage of any opportunity that came their way.

2. Programs and living units at the Paso Robles School were traditionally named by the superintendent after nearby cities and communities. Escalon is a small town.

3. Not that there is anything wrong with custody and control. An oft quoted axiom is, "You can't treat them if they're not there." It should have a corollary, though: "Just keeping them there isn't treating them."

4. We did have one little problem with these rooms. Each one had its own toilet, connected to the sewer system by a T-joint that also tied in, through the wall, with the toilet of an adjacent room. Why this particular building was plumbed with T-joints, I'll never know. Perhaps the plumber drank. At any rate, the result was that the flushing of one toilet shot part of its contents down the sewer, and the other part straight across into the toilet next door. This, of course, called for retaliation. On numerous occasions, wards would stay up the greater part of the night, shouting curses and flushing toilets at each other through the

walls. We eventually achieved a cease-fire, not through group therapy as you might imagine, but by replacing the T-joints with Y-joints.

5. No small order, but nonetheless the necessary characteristics of a truly effective youth worker in a correctional treatment program.

6. Among those suggestions he didn't approve were mud baths, parachute jumping, and group masturbation.

7. Some wards gained much simply from being exposed to *new experience*. One such youth from a high delinquency ghetto had been committed to the State for stabbing a rival gang member with a knife had never in his life been fishing. While returning from one such excursion, he was overheard remarking in all sincerity to a companion, "Gee, I didn't know you could have such kicks without breaking the law."

8. Taken from "Paso Robles Pioneer Treatment Program," *California Youth Authority Quarterly*, Winter, 1957, pp. 8-9.

9. While I do not view the medical model as very useful in working with delinquents, I used the term "patients" several times in this early article, partly because I was at that time overly impressed with my hospital training and experience. But, additionally, I wanted to shake up the thinking of Youth Authority staff who perceived wards as adversaries, rather than as people needing help.

10. "Permissive" in the sense of open communication of feelings and problems—not in the sense of permitting uncontrolled or antisocial behavior.

11. Adding "mother figures"—female youth workers—would also be valuable. (This has since been done in every Youth Authority facility.)

12. For a discussion of this therapeutic teaching approach, see Lewis, William B., and Gunn, Alex M., "Classroom Counseling of the Delinquent," *California Youth Authority Quarterly*, Summer 1959, pp. 16-18.

13. Technically, psychotics were supposed to be under the care of the Department of Mental Hygiene, not the Youth Authority. But often it did not work that way. Mental Hygiene was loathe to accept juvenile delinquent psychotics.

Chapter VIII

Correctional Counseling:
What, Why, How Much, and Who?

WHAT

When the man on the street thinks of "counseling," he usually has in mind a person who needs to go to an expert for technical advice — usually for a fee. That is not the kind of counseling we are concerned with in the treatment of delinquent youth. There are, to be sure, dozens of kinds of technical counseling, each of which may be useful to a given institutionalized youthful offender at certain times, in resolving specific problems. Just a few of the adjectives used to specify types of counseling are religious, educational, legal, medical, financial, premarital, marital, postmarital, vocational, vacational, and "income taxical." None of these is correctional counseling. Then what IS?

"Correctional Counseling," hereafter referred to as just plain "counseling," consists of *ongoing*, positive, interpersonal relationships as the vehicle through which a variety of systematic verbal techniques can be applied to increase the counselee's *feelings* of self-satisfaction, *and* improve his *actual* social adjustments.

A counselor, then, following up on this definition, is a person who, first, has learned how to establish growth-inducing interpersonal relationships (meet needs and serve as an ego model). Second, he has learned some specialized verbal techniques through which he can help the counselee to focus on pertinent areas of development and problem solving. His major contributions in a residential treatment setting are (1) the direct application of these skills to improving the self-concepts and social effectiveness of the residents, *and* (2) the training and supervision of other staff in the development of their own interpersonal and verbal counseling abilities.

WHY AND HOW MUCH?

Recall, from our earlier discussion of self-concept, that an individual develops self-awareness — gets to know who he is — through his relationships with other people. If these relationships have been sparse, at too few levels of intimacy, or have been destructive instead of growth-supporting, then the individual's social-emotional adjustment may be fouled up in two general ways. He may be trapped in a tiny, impoverished world of interpersonal experience, and a drab, boring existence; or he may be chronically at war with many of the persons and groups who make up his interpersonal world, no matter how simple or complex it is, so that his life is continually plagued by conflict and stress. Both of these conditions are common among juvenile delinquents. Undirected groping about, seeking a more meaningful, stimulating existence (looking for "kicks"), and lashing out aggressively against the world in response to interpersonal frustration and pain are, indeed, two major sources of delinquent behavior.

In contrast to the stunted or distorted self-images, and the boring or conflict ridden lifestyles of many delinquents, a mature, emotionally and socially well-integrated person enjoys a solid, pleasing sense of self, with roots in a broad range of satisfying interpersonal experiences. He is confident of his identity, and can operate effectively as an individual in intimate, one-to-one relationships; in small, close groups such as a family, and in a great variety of increasingly large and less intimate groups, such as social clubs, service organizations, trades and professions, church denominations, ethnic groups, and the human race.

A major objective of a counseling program for delinquent youth is to help them expand themselves — to encourage the development of a satisfying sense of identity, and the ability to function effectively in a variety of interpersonal situations and at several different levels on the intimacy continuum. It follows then, that an adequate counseling *program* must include more than the opportunity to be periodically chewed out by, or shoot the breeze with, a staff member. Instead, it must provide (in addition to one shot "crisis counseling" for problems which arise unpredictably) organized, scheduled, ongoing counseling sessions to promote self-discovery, and interpersonal growth *at several levels of intimacy.* As an arbitrary minimum, ongoing counseling should be made available (1) on an individual basis to promote self-discovery in an intimate, one-to-one relationship; (2) in a small group setting to help certain youths find out what its like to belong to a small, relatively intimate "family substitute" which communicates openly within itself, and whose members care about, and try to help each other; and (3) in large, total living unit meetings which permit the growth of self-image as a member of a community, sharing in its benefits, and responsible to the other members for "carrying one's load" — for contributing to the welfare of the community as a whole.

If a residential treatment program includes sufficient competent counseling services at the three levels of intimacy suggested as minimal;[1] the participating youths reap the following benefits, all potent agents in the growth process we seek to advance:

A. A legitimate setting which permits discharge of angry or painful feelings, lowers tension levels and forestalls many uncontrolled behavioral outbursts. Introduction of an adequate counseling program to a residential program, in every instance in my experience, has produced a dramatic reduction in incidents of violence and other antisocial acts. Counseling is not only a treatment tool. It is an effective management device.

B. The "ego model" behavior of the counselor forces the collapse of the delinquent's stereotyped view of adults as authoritarian, hostile, rejecting, demanding, or uncaring creeps.

C. Troubled people often assume that they are the only ones on earth plagued by such problems. They feel isolated, lost, and sometimes ashamed. These feelings, paralyzing their growth potential, can be relieved through observing firsthand in a counseling (especially group) program that others share similar problems.

D. Low self-esteem is elevated through being treated as a worthy human being with valuable ideas and opinions.

E. Inappropriate, self-defeating behavior is often based on a false notion of how others see us. Counseling can provide the delinquent youth information as to how he *really* appears to others, and how his own behavior and comments effect them.[2]

F. In his search for new levels of identity, the delinquent needs non-threatening situations in which he can "try on for size" new ways of relating to others — new roles and interpersonal behaviors. He can find out by actual test how they work, how they "fit" him, and whether or not they produce satisfying results. An adequate counseling program provides such laboratories.

G. This is a kind of extension of (F) above. A counseling program which includes the minimal three levels of intimacy (one-to-one; small group; and large group — the entire living unit population) will provide a good variety of testing grounds for experimenting with new social roles and styles. But it is really not enough. The residential program remains a kind of artificial world. Any new, improved concepts, attitudes and social skills acquired within it must be transferable to the world of reality outside if they are to be worth anything to the delinquent* when he leaves. While still on the inside, he needs the opportunity to interact with members of the outside social world — his own family, other significant people in his life, volunteers. Even informal, non-counseling contacts with the community "out there" — unstructured family visits, volunteer-sponsored recreational events, athletic events with nearby public schools — provide the youth real-life testing grounds for the new attitudes and behaviors he is acquiring through the counseling program. Additionally, frequent contact with people from the outside community helps to humanize and normalize the institutional living program.

H. Counseling interaction with a variety of types of people — the opposite sex, different ethnic groups, persons of diverse

---

*Or, hopefully, the ex-delinquent, or at least the not-as-delinquent.

backgrounds and customs — permits the delinquent youth to expand his awareness of the social world around him, and identify himself with it.

WHO

Correctional counselors may come to the job armed with appropriate skills acquired through formal education.[1] Most do not, and must learn these skills through on-the-job training by competent counselors. There aren't enough professionally trained counselors available to make a dent in the surface of the institutionalized youth population. Consequently, paraprofessional counselors, trained on the job, must carry the bulk of the load if needed services are to be delivered. As a matter of fact, such persons, once trained can often out perform their trainers. Some ex-offenders and ex-drug abusers, for example, are easier for delinquent youths to identify with. They can provide more relevant counseling than can many professionals who have led more sheltered lives.

Every institution or group residence for delinquents ought to have a trained and experienced professional in charge of its overall counseling program.

Ideally, this counseling program supervisor should be trained in counseling, group work, social work, psychology or related field. In a relatively small facility, this supervisor would personally train and supervise available staff in the theory and techniques of counseling. In a larger facility, *each living unit* should have its own resident counselor. His duties, in addition to counseling per se, would include the ongoing training and supervision of the staff on his unit in counseling skills. This position could be filled either by a person with a degree in an appropriate field, plus training and ongoing supervision by the counseling program supervisor, or by someone with less formal education and more on-the-job training and counseling experience.

Formal education requirements for counseling program supervisors and counselors should never be so ironclad as to prevent the hiring and promotion of persons with human relations and counseling skills acquired through nonuniversity experiences. One of the finest, most competent counselors with delinquent youth I have had

the pleasure to train was a man whose credentials were a high
school diploma and twenty years experience as a bartender.[4]

Counseling versus Psychotherapy

Untold hours have been wasted by counselors and psychotherapists arguing about what constitutes psychotherapy *as opposed to
counseling.* They rarely reach any sensible conclusions because
they are starting with a false premise. Therapy is *not* opposed to
counseling. They are not discrete phenomena that can be neatly
packed into two separate boxes. They are basically the same
thing—application of systematic verbal (and sometimes nonverbal)
techniques, through the medium of a positive interpersonal relationship, to produce greater happiness and actual social effectiveness in
the counselee.

Persons who are all hung up with the need to dichotomize therapy
and counseling usually call *themselves* "therapists." Through jeal-
ously guarding this *word*, they can keep reminding the world (and
themselves) that they know a lot more than other folks, especially
counselors, without having to come right out and brag about it.

Most attempts to separate personality counseling and therapy into
two distinct categories are based on criteria such as complexity of
theory and techniques used, or "depth" of material discussed. Any
such separation has to be arbitrary and artificial, because these factors form a continuum, ranging from very simple, or very shallow,
to very complex, or very deep. All degrees of complexity or
"depth" exist in between. It's like saying that an ocean is really
two separate things—a deep sea and a shallow sea. But where—at
what absolute point—does the shallow sea end and the deep sea
begin?

Another common vanity-based approach to differentiation between therapy and counseling is to define the process as either one
or the other, depending upon the profession of whoever is doing it.
These customs have changed as newer professions have evolved
from stepchild status toward wider acceptance. For a long time,
only psychiatrists (MD) could claim to do therapy. Psychologists
could do counseling. Nowadays, thanks to professional organizations and public image work, psychologists, social workers, and

other classes have gained recognition as therapists. They are still doing about the same things they used to do, but can call it therapy now. Really, now, isn't this whole business kind of silly? The function can't logically be defined on the basis of the name, or class, of the person doing the functioning. If a graduate welder is engaged in sawing boards and nailing them together to make a house frame, must we say he is welding?

One more point on this issue, counseling versus therapy, and we will move on. Whether you call yourself a counselor or a therapist* you should proceed with caution in adding new (to you) techniques to your practice with real, live people. Remember that your primary goal is to help your counselee. If you use him as a laboratory, to experiment blindly with techniques you don't understand yourself, you may confuse him and damage him. Innovation, though necessary to progress, is most meaningful when we have a sound knowledge of what we are innovating upon. Read, study, and seek ongoing training and supervision from more experienced counselors. Learn to recognize your own limits (which will expand) of skill and understanding, and to seek consultation when you approach them.

EGO PATCHING AT THE ONE-TO-ONE LEVEL OF INTIMACY: INDIVIDUAL COUNSELING — HOW DO YOU DO IT?

No simple cookbook answer to this question is possible. The purpose of this book is *not* to present a comprehensive survey of the theories and methods of personality counseling. This has already been done by a number of far more scholarly writers than I. Yet I can't do what I want to do — share with you some methods of counseling that I have found to *work* with delinquents — without referring first to some other theories and methods. The reason I can't is that nobody ever invents a new, unique method. We only discover new ways to combine and integrate principles that already exist. Newton didn't *invent* the law of gravity. Things didn't fall upward before he made the scene. The law has been around since creation.

---

*Or clinician, or caseworker, or whatever.

But Newton combined his unique personal observations with existing historical knowledge to create a fresh perspective from which this law could be recognized and defined.

Another way to put this is that the methods I have tried, tested, rearranged, and evolved into forms that work with delinquents, are stolen.* This kind of thievery doesn't embarrass me though, because the people whose concepts are incorporated in my counseling philosophy and style went through the same process in reaching *their* individual vistas and systems.

With a salute, then, to all those famous and infamous people whose ideas have shaped and reshaped my viewpoint and treatment strategies with delinquents, let's get on with the business at hand — one-to-one headstuffing.

To reduce youths' delinquent behavior, personality counseling must do two things: help them find out who they are (enrich and strengthen self-concepts), and stimulate the growth of their ability to analyze reality and predict consequences of their own behaviors (patching holes in their egos). I do this by meeting their emotional needs in the counseling relationship (thereby becoming an ego model), and by employing verbal and auxiliary techniques specifically designed to focus on identity problems and encourage "ego exercise" — active practice in *using* their developing reality-testing and decision-making gear.[5]

Delinquents come with a variety of levels of social maturity, need deprivation patterns, verbal skills, and clusters of adjunctive, nondelinquency personality problems. No single technique of counseling is going to be effective with all of them. A counselor who is steeped in one school of treatment theory and skilled only in its techniques will find that he can work effectively with only a minor segment of the delinquent population — those individuals whose level of maturity, sophistication, verbal skill, and problem clusters happen to fit his one theory and technique.

A corollary to this statement is that the more schools of thought

---

*Or at best, discovered. Sort of like Columbus' "discovery" of America, much to the surprise of all those Indians who thought they already knew it was here.

and counseling techniques a counselor is well versed in, the more armament he has at his disposal for working effectively with diverse types of individuals.

One delinquent may be helped to find out who he is and improve the accuracy of his perception of reality through analyzing early life experiences and relating these to present attitudes, behaviors, social strategies, and defenses. Another may not be able to dig all this fancy stuff, and can best find out who he is (and expand upon it) by measuring his muscles in an ongoing weight training program in front of a full length mirror under the tutelage of an interested, patient, encouraging, weight lifting-oriented counselor — ego model. Still others (in my opinion, most) may enhance their self-understanding and strengthen their reality-testing most effectively through discovering the basic, legitimate human needs underlying their symptomatic behaviors and finding ways to satisfy these needs. I refer to this particular approach as *"Why Not?"* Therapy, and will subsequently illustrate it.

Many other treatment strategies and techniques have been defined and developed. With a large repertoire at his disposal, a counselor can approach individuals with techniques best suited to their specific personalities. Further, he can shift emphasis and techniques to match new developments in the course of each individual's progress.

In the chapters that follow, some of these counseling strategies will be illustrated. We will meet a number of seriously maladapted, delinquent young men, and take a look at what goes on in a psychologist's office — or at least some of the things that *went* on in *this* psychologist's office.

These cases were chosen from my files on the basis that they were, in general, considered poor candidates for verbal treatment by usual standards. Many of them had been turned down as "non-amenable" to therapy in other settings. Others had been tried with less flexible approaches (e.g., classical analytic therapy), and either got nothing out of it or got worse.

Counseling effectively with a variety of individuals requires a variety of strategies and methods, and the sensitivity to know (feel?) when to apply which. Some of them (for example, the hypnoanalytic techniques) require extensive training. Their use is even restricted by law in many places to specified professional classes. Others, not so dramatic, but useful with a wider range of counselees (for example, recognition and reflecting of feelings) suffer no such restrictions and may be practiced by anyone who learns how.[6]

In the following case reviews, I will attempt to clarify the strategies and techniques as we go along. Don't forget that first priority in developing an effective correctional treatment program does *not* go to formal counseling services. It goes to the everyday interpersonal environment, or atmosphere, in which counseling, education, recreation, and the other program elements are expected to function. None of the formal elements can consistently produce growth in a setting dominated by cold, apathetic, inconsistent, or punitive staff attitudes and leadership styles.

In a wholesome interpersonal atmosphere, the ordinary, day-to-day living experiences can produce positive personality changes. In a dehumanized environment, formal counseling efforts will be doomed to failure before they are begun.

NOTES

1. Ideally, these should be supplemented by a variety of treatment-oriented activity groups offering even more opportunities for discovering new facets of the self. Each teacher, coach, stamp collectors' club supervisor, music instructor, or regularly visiting volunteer is a potential ego-model who could learn to integrate counseling techniques into his specialty activities.

2. We will dig into some group counseling methods later. One chapter will describe, and illustrate with case material, a group technique specifically designed to produce growth through correcting false ideas of how others see us and react to us.

3. They will soon learn, however, that they are not fully armed; that a lot of the knowledge acquired in a university is unrelated to the real, everyday world; and that corrective feedback in a practice setting is necessary before their knowledge becomes very useful in working with delinquent youths.

4. When you think about it, the human relations skills a bartender has to develop to survive — calming hostile drunks and listening compassionately to weepy ones — may be more appropriate background for a professional counseling career than the stuff taught in the universities.

5. These auxiliary techniques often involve the use of very concrete tools such

as weights, tape measures, mirrors, tape recorders or videotape. My aim is to help youths come to grips with their underdeveloped self-images and discover, or develop, previously unrecognized facets of themselves.

6. Some of these techniques are also useful in everyday conversations and interpersonal transactions outside the counseling setting. They can make you an improved conversationalist.

Chapter IX

Withdrawn Willie Comes Alive —
"Why Not?" Therapy:
Counseling with
a Schizoid Exhibitionist

"Why Not?" Counseling is my adaptation of a system called "need integrative therapy" by Vance K. Boileau.[1]

I was immediately attracted to this system because it tied in closely with my own observations on the important roles that self-concept (or lack of it) and incomplete ego development play in fostering delinquency. Recall that the self-concept and development of the ego (reality-testing ability) are products of how well, and under what conditions, the basic, legitimate, human needs were satisfied during the individual's developmental years.

Traditional analytic therapists tend to focus on past history, or its consequent current interpersonal defenses and strategies. They point out to the patient that times have changed, assuming that when the patient recognizes ("gains insight") that his present troublesome behavior is based on childhood events or conditions which no longer exist, he will recognize how stupid he is, and stop behaving that way. With many, many delinquents, this approach doesn't work. They accept the therapist's interpretations all right, but use them to justify their delinquency instead of overcoming it. ("Well of course I'm a burglar. I'm seeking the affection my mother denied me. It's her fault, so what can I do about it?") "Why Not? Counseling," by comparison, takes the position that every delinquent act (or other personality symptom) is somebody's screwed-up attempt to satisfy an underlying *legitimate* human need. The task is not to convince the counselee how screwed up he is, but rather:

1. To identify the legitimate need underlying his symptom, and differentiate between it and the goals which are not his own, but have been imposed on him by someone else. (Who says you have to . . . ?)
2. To present the legitimate need directly to his own ego for evaluation as to whether it is a good or bad need. (Is there something the matter with . . . ?)
3. When he recognizes the legitimacy of his need, to present directly to his ego the question of whether or not the symptomatic behavior is working — is it really gaining the need satisfaction he is seeking? (Is this method you've been using getting you . . . ?)
4. When he recognizes that his present disguised attempt to satisfy the need is not working, to present to his ego the question, "Might there be some other approaches to getting what you want that *will* work?"
5. To help him identify alternative approaches to pursuing the gratification of the need, and prod his ego toward a decision to try one or more of the alternatives to see if they work. (Youth: "Gee, I wonder if that would work. I wonder if I dare try it?" Counselor: "*Why not?* What have you got to lose?")

What he's got to lose is his symptom, because when he finds a way to *directly* satisfy the underlying legitimate need, the screwed-up, disguised attempt to satisfy it no longer has a purpose, and it is discarded.

Now, let's meet Withdrawn Willie, an emotionally flat, socially isolated young man, committed to the Youth Authority for repeated episodes of exhibiting his penis in public. Willie's individual counseling program consisted of one session per week for twelve weeks, at which time we terminated the interviews by mutual agreement on the grounds that we had made maximum progress in improving Willie's self-concept, reality-testing and social effectiveness, and he had been recommended for parole.

The first three sessions of Willie's counseling series, edited from my notes (written up immediately after each interview), illustrate the "Why Not?" approach to counseling, and especially, how it can be used to counteract the harmful effects of earlier "therapy" of a traditional type. Willie had experienced several months of analytic therapy before being paroled from another institution, and, as we shall see, used it to *rationalize and perpetuate* his antisocial behavior. Consequently, he became a parole violator a few weeks after his release. He had been in the Paso Robles institution for several months, withdrawn, not communicating, not participating in program—vegetating—when he came to my attention.

In the pessimistic words of the social worker who interviewed Willie as a staff-referred candidate for treatment:

> Willie is a slenderly built 16-year-old with pleasant physical features which could be enhanced by a mien of self-confidence, and thereby become an asset to him. He gives the impression of being physically weak and completely lacking in zest, of hiding away, but of being capable of a substantially fuller grasp on things if he had an idea where to start. The boy's intelligence level appears less than average with verbal material. Variations between his IQ scores are sufficient to cause us to wonder if re-testing would be appropriate. Willie was friendly but maintained a detached attitude. He expressed more of what he has been told from various sources than any feelings or concepts essentially his own.
>
> The boy's primary interest in therapy at the interview was to "tell someone where I want to live when I leave here." . . .
>
> Some attempt at treatment should be undertaken. It would seem to involve a long term process for anything other than minimal gain. A strong supportive identification figure, who would aid Willie to formulate or strengthen a positive concept of himself within an appropriate value system, would seem essential if this boy is to learn how to grow up. He does not appear to be a particularly good candidate for psychotherapy . . .

Okay, let's find out.

SESSION #1 NOTES

Willie presented himself in a shy, limp, half-smiling way which suggested he would like to be friendly, but isn't sure how, or if he is brave enough to try. I asked what he hoped to get from meeting with me. He said he hoped to learn to get along better with people his age, describing himself as a "loner." I asked, "Who says you have to be a social butterfly? Is there anything wrong with keeping to yourself?"[2] After puzzling a few moments, Willie responded that he didn't see anything illegal about staying to himself, and that he *doesn't* have to mix, but that he honestly feels he is missing out on something because he can't express himself when the other guys are talking about things. I said, "Sometimes you really want to say something in those conversations, and feel you have something good to say, but you are afraid to do it. You just can't push yourself into the stream of things."[3] Willie sighed his affirmation. (Note to self for probable future use: Willie's needs for more aggressive self-presentation, and probably a great underlying acceptance hunger.)

I asked Willie to tell me about why he is locked up. He blandly stated that he exposed himself to girls, but quickly added that his problem is now under control. I asked what he was trying to do when he exposed himself. (Here I was seeking clues as to the legitimate needs underlying the symptom.) He glibly replied that he was hoping to have intercourse with the girls he exposed himself to. I laughed, and asked if he seriously believed that those strange girls on public streets would suddenly come upon a stranger with his penis out and volunteer for intercourse on the spot. (Encouraging reality testing.)

Willie grinned. I asked, "What would you do if you were walking down the sidewalk, and suddenly a strange woman came up to you, pulled up her skirt and aimed her naked sex organ at you? Would you feel romantically inclined and take her on right there?" Willie blushed, stammered, laughed, and blurted, "I'd probably run like hell!" I laughed with him, and then continued, "Okay. That's pretty silly. You weren't seriously trying to drum up some sexual intercourse. I wonder what you *were* after. What *did* you want in those situations?" (Still looking for the underlying needs.)

Willie thought seriously, looking puzzled. "I don't know. I just wanted 'em to look at me, I guess." "Okay. Let's start with that. It seems pretty obvious that if you show something to somebody, you want them to look at it. Now, can we go a step further? *How* did you want them to look at you? Was there any special way you wanted them to look at you? Any special way you wanted them to feel?" Willie sat silently for a few moments, then mumbled, "I don't know. I guess I wanted them to be excited or something." "What do you mean 'excited'?"

This line of questioning shortly led to my identification of Willie's wish-to-be-admired as an important legitimate need underlying his exhibitionistic acts. "Okay," I pursued the issue, "You would say, then, that you wanted these girls to look at you and admire you, or approve of you. Is that right?" Willie nodded vigorously, concurring. I asked, "Is there something wrong with wanting to be looked at with admiration or approval?" Willie churned the question, and concluded that, indeed, there is nothing wrong with wanting to be admired by members of the opposite sex—a conclusion which I supported by noting that most men like to look good to women. I continued, "Since there is nothing wrong with your wanting to be looked at with admiration and approval—this is a normal human desire— all we have to ask is how effective is this approach of yours, exposing yourself, at getting what you want?" He pondered, finally mumbling, "Not very good." I said, "You got half of what you wanted." He said, sheepishly, "Yeah. I got looked at."

Feeling that Willie had received all the ego exercise he could handle for one day, I closed the session, which lasted only thirty-five minutes, by suggesting that, as time goes by, perhaps we can discuss some ways of getting admiration and approval that *will* work, and won't get him in jail either. We agreed to meet once a week. (The reader will notice that "Why Not?" counseling gets down to issues in a hurry. Little, if any, time is spent in this approach on excursions into childhood memories, elaborate analysis of defenses, interpretation of fantasies and the like.)

SESSION #2 NOTES

I reviewed what we covered last time regarding Willie's sex offenses, the underlying legitimate need for attention *with* admiration and approval, and the conclusion that the exhibitionistic acts were not effective in satisfying that need. We then explored a bit further, identifying a need for sexual excitement also underlying his acts. We questioned, and affirmed with his ego, the legitimacy of having sexual urges. Then I introduced the idea that many modes of satisfying sexual urges are possible, and they are not all of equal personal and social acceptability.[4] Willie resisted this concept, assuring me that his sex problem was solved — he could just get along without sex by keeping busy with other things. I pushed the issue, challenging his position with questions, such as, "Can you see any possible differences in consequences between, say, masturbating in private and exposing your penis in public?" He sidestepped the question, commenting at first that he didn't see anything wrong with masturbating, and that he didn't believe the stories about it ". . . messing up your body and stuff," but added that he is planning to try to quit it. I asked why, if he didn't think it wrong or harmful. He then refuted his first comment, saying that maybe masturbating is what makes him skinny and behind in his school work.

I took time out from the exchange to provide some information that Willie needed as preparation for further exploration of his sexual self-concept. I explained that there is no known physical harm done by masturbation, and pointed out that physiological processes leading to sexual climax through masturbation and heterosexual intercourse are identical. If the physical process of masturbating to climax makes people go crazy, then all married couples who have sexual intercourse regularly, should be crazy too.* Willie absorbed this information with great interest, and said that it made sense to him.

"Okay," I continued, "The physical act of masturbation is not known to be harmful in itself. But attitudes *about* masturbation can cause trouble — worry, guilt, and other disturbed feelings. These *can* be harmful."

Willie then told me how uncomfortable he feels when others kid around, talking about sex, perhaps teasing someone about being caught masturbating. I asked him for further description of these uncomfortable feelings. He explained that he, himself, has masturbated, and that the ridicule really applies to him as well as the other guy, if the group only knew, and that they would dislike him and

---

*Some of them are, but probably for other reasons.

not associate with him if they ". . . did know I did it or if they knew what I am in here for."

First, I asked Willie how many of the other guys in that group had masturbated. He laughed and said, "All of them, probably." Then I asked, "Do they really dislike and stone out* this guy they are kidding about being caught?" Willie said, "No. They just kid him." I said, "It would be kind of strange if they really disliked him for doing something they know they all do." He concurred. Then (still pressing Willie to exercise his ego – to learn to discriminate between different kinds of sex acts and circumstances) I asked, "Is the same thing true for exposing your penis to girls on the street?" He saw the difference and said that the group *really would* dislike him, and would not want to associate with him if they knew about *that*.

At this point, I switched the focus back to his need for approval, pointing out that first we had discovered how important it was to him to be noticed and approved by girls, and now he had been talking about wanting to be accepted and approved by his buddies. I asked again if there was anything wrong with wanting to be noticed, liked, and approved of. He said, "No." Then, I pointed out that it was not his sex urges per se, nor even, some kinds of active sex behavior, such as private masturbation, that deprived him of this desired social approval. Rather, it was the *kind* of sexual behavior, and the *circumstances* under which it occurred that seemed to affect how people thought of him. Willie nodded his understanding.

Just before the end of the session, Willie commented out of a clear blue sky, that he thinks he sometimes tries to blame other people and events for his troubles. He gave some illustrations, and implied that he has not been giving proper blame to his own decisions in bringing difficulties upon himself. I commented that it's a good thing his own decisions had something to do with his troubles. This meant that he could also make decisions which would bring better consequences, whereas if his problems were "caused" by the uncle who sexually molested him when Willie was a small child, or by his having to live in the city of Fresno – well, it would be kind of hard now to go back and change that uncle, or the city.

---

*"Stone Out" is delinquentese for "ostracize."

SESSION #3 NOTES

I asked Willie where he would like to begin today. He replied that he has been doing a lot of thinking about what I said about masturbation, and it ". . . makes a lot of sense." "How's that?" I asked. He said that it just makes a lot more sense than a lot of things people have told him about it in the past (the fear and guilt-provoking myths we discussed last time). Willie's emotional tone accompanying these comments carried an air of relief. This context soon permitted me to summarize the principle that sex hunger is just that, a physical hunger which can be attached to any number of specific appetites, just as stomach pang hunger can be attached to specific appetites for steak, for pizza, for pistachio ice cream, or a variety of other foods.

Society doesn't much care what foods you select to appease your stomach, but your sexual menu is another matter. Society has set up rules and laws, not about having sex hunger, but about how you may satisfy it — which specific appetites you may or may not feed. Some appetites are fully approved — for example, face to face intercourse between husband and wife. Others, such as masturbation in private, are quietly condoned. Still others, such as appetites for rape, sex with children, or exhibiting your penis in public, will invariably bring the wrath of society down upon you. The trick is, since there are many possible ways to satisfy the sex urge (which we already agreed is a normal and healthy need), to pick out ways that both get the job done (are satisfying) and don't get you in trouble. Willie listened to this intently, nodding his agreement. Following my little dissertation on sex appetites, Willie remained silent for some time, apparently having pursued that subject as far as he cared to.

I inquired (still exploring his need pattern) how he felt about being locked up. The gist of his response was that he rather likes being in the institution, perceiving it as a miniature community with components parallel to those of the real world — ". . . school, work, movies." He does feel somewhat deprived of contact with girls, and of freedom of choice as to when and where to come and go. Being a "loner," however, and ". . . able to adjust wherever I am," these deprivations are not unbearable. I said, "Well, you miss these things, but not much more than you did on the outs. You didn't have them there either.'' He agreed, with one exception. He told me about a girl cousin who used to go to the movies with him, hold hands, and share some pleasant feelings of romance. I suggested that if he saw a chance of enjoying more close relationships with people, especially girls, ''on the outs,'' he might see a bigger difference between that and life in an institution. He agreed that that would make a big difference.

I asked Willie, since he feels this need for closeness with others, why he chooses to be a ''loner,'' as he describes himself. At first he said that he was happy as a loner, but quickly reduced this claim to another statement of his ability to ''adjust'' to whatever fate hands him — to tolerate it without fuss and furor. Then he blamed his uncle for never letting him bring his friends home, being ashamed of their meager trailer court home. He would meet friends, visit at their homes, then, being unable to repay the courtesy, would ''. . . throw them for a shine'' (ignore them). I pointed out that, while his uncle may have kept him from bringing friends into their home, it was *Willie*, not the uncle, who made the decision to drop his new friends and not carry on friendly relationships outside the home.

At this point Willie commented, ''When I *really* started throwing people for a shine was when my grandmother died.'' He went on to describe a fairly close relationship with her, and guilt feelings he experienced after her death (for having not always made life easy for her). He pointed out that he had not cried when she went to the hospital, while others, including his brother, had cried, which made Willie feel guilty when she died. I acknowledged these feelings but asked where all of this was leading us. Willie responded with a cut and dried psychoanalytic type formulation, apparently ''learned'' in his earlier experience in therapy. The gist of this ''insight,'' was, according to Willie, that he had ''blamed'' himself for his grandmother's death and drove himself into isolation (became a loner) and got himself into trouble with the law in order to punish himself.

I challenged this pat formula, ''Oh, how did you cause her death?'' He backtracked hastily, assuring me that he really didn't cause her death, but ''. . . I just kind of blamed myself for it somehow.'' I asked, ''Why would you want to do that? You either caused her death in some way, or you didn't. If you didn't, why would you want to blame yourself? I don't understand.'' Under this kind of questioning, Willie's rational ego shifted into gear, and he clarified how the situation really was between his grandmother and him — some good, some bad; some kindness, some meanness on both sides. We agreed that his ''. . . blaming myself for her death'' was not an accurate description of his reaction, which, in fact, consisted of feeling guilty about not having treated her better when he had the chance — a normal and usual reaction to a loved one's death.

I pointed out additionally that his grandmother's death could not, and did not, *make* him isolate himself or commit crimes. He may have felt sad and guilty about it all right, but those feelings did not *make* him an isolate, nor get him locked up. Rather, it was the *action* he *decided* to take in response to these feelings that brought on the trouble. Feelings, even irrational feelings, can get us into trouble only when we translate them into ineffective or self-defeating actions. Willie pondered these concepts seriously, nodding affirmation.

At this point I suggested that we back up and take a look at this recipe — grandmother's death — self-blame — punishment seeking — isolation — crime — from a different angle.* I led Willie through a re-discussion of this same material, this time with questions and comments aimed at focusing on the legitimate needs underlying his symptomatic behavior.

We discovered that, following his grandmother's death, Willie felt guilty and was angry at himself for not having been nicer to her. I pointed out, therefore, that what he really wanted was to be able to think of himself as a person who is nice, kind, considerate and loving, rather than a mean, bad one. He agreed. I asked if there was anything wrong with that. There wasn't. In fact, Willie thought that wanting to see oneself as a good, kind person was a downright commendable need. Having determined the nature and acceptability of the need, I said, ''Well then, we have to ask now about how

---

*Note in what follows how the ''Why Not?,'' or need evaluation, approach can be used to overcome rationalizations previously implanted by more traditional ''therapy,'' and at the same time help the counselee toward a clearer understanding of his own legitimate needs and the ineffectiveness of his symptomatic behavior in gaining need satisfaction.

effective were your methods of trying to satisfy it." Willie was able to conclude that isolating himself socially and exposing his penis in public were not especially good ways of making him see himself as a more kind, considerate, loving person. In fact, these behaviors led to the reverse, even more loathesome self-picture. I asked if he could think of any ways that might work to get him what he wanted. He said, "Yep. Talk to people and be nice to them." "Okay, Willie, *why not* try it and see if it works?" "Okay, maybe I will."

Willie tried it, and it worked. Over the next nine weeks, while we discussed further his needs and methods of satisfying them, living unit staff reported remarkable changes in his social behavior. Withdrawn Willie came alive, not only mixing freely as a participant in informal bull sessions, but contributing often and constructively as a member of the living unit community in the regularly scheduled large group meetings. About a year after his parole, Willie wrote to me, proudly, to let me know that he was making progress in school, was bowling in a league, and had a girlfriend.

NOTES

1. Boileau, Vance K. "New Techniques in Brief Psychotherapy." *Psychological Reports*, 1958, *4*, 627-645.

2. A major difference in strategy between "why not?" and traditional therapy is that the counselor does not automatically assume that everything the counselee thinks is bad about himself is, in reality, bad. Maybe society is making unrealistic demands upon him, and convincing him that perfectly legitimate behaviors are bad. The "Why Not?" counselor actively challenges the traditional assumption by asking the counselee's ego to determine whether the problem is indeed his, or is it society's.

3. This kind of response, called a "reflection" — listening to the feeling and thoughts expressed and demonstrating that you are interested and understanding by re-phrasing and uncritically reflecting them back to the counselee — is extremely useful in almost any counseling setting. It has the effect of neutralizing feelings that block communications and stimulating forward progress in the counselee's self-exploration. The reflection technique was developed by Carl Rogers. Remember the term "reflecting." It will be used often in later chapters.

4. Strangely, but commonly, juvenile sex offenders see sex as an all or none proposition. They fail to recognize that different social sanctions are placed on different modes of expression. The most frequent solution proposed by these youths for their various sexual deviation problems is giving up sex altogether. They really believe that total abstinence or get-in-trouble are the only possible

alternatives. They deeply believe they are doomed because they won't be able to abstain forever, although they will say they can, and plan to do so, and everything will be rosy as they lead their non-sexual lives, keeping busy and doing lots of push-ups. Unless this attitude is altered they will fail, of course. They soon find themselves doing their push-ups with no hands, and are driven to find a sexual outlet — usually the deviant one they are used to.

Chapter X

Heinous Harry:
An Unsocialized Exploder
Finds Out Who He Is

Fifteen-year-old Harry Cromwell was introduced in Chapter VII. My first client in the Youth Authority, the seriousness of his emotional problems pointed up the need for a specialized program for such disturbed youths. Harry triggered the development of Escalon, the prototype specialized treatment program in the Youth Authority.

In addition to Harry's historical role in the development of the Youth Authority's subsequent treatment facilities, his therapy in itself was clinically noteworthy. It illustrated how drawing the human figure may be used as an adjunct to bogged down verbal therapy, and demonstrated with remarkable clarity how the struggle for a satisfying self-image may be projected onto the drawing. Perhaps the most interesting aspect of this series of drawings lies in its illustration of how art may be used as a means of estimating progress in psychotherapy.

Harry had been well known to local police since he was ten years old. He had been involved in repeated runaways, petty thefts, curfew violations, and other minor offenses. He was committed to the California Youth Authority for auto theft at the age of fourteen. After nine months at the Paso Robles School for Boys, Harry ran away (stealing two more cars in the process). He had just been apprehended and returned to the institution in a raging, distraught, almost incoherent state, when he was brought to the attention of the writer, who was at that time the institution's new clinical psychologist.

An excerpt from Harry's initial psychological evaluation reveals:

. . . an acute shortage of intellectual controls in this boy's emotional life. Use of fantasy is meager and immature, so that he must depend largely upon repression and the avoidance of external emotional stimuli to keep from being overwhelmed by his impulses. These defenses are only partially effective, and he cannot permanently avoid his own impulse life, so emotional energy is stored for a period, swelling and growing, until it bursts through the fragile defenses and spills out in a flood of uncontrolled emotional behavior.

Beneath this alternately apathetic and volatile emotionality lies a personality structure which, while shrunken and scarred by affectional deprivation, is fairly well intact. There is still some capacity for forming meaningful relationships and identifications, under permissive circumstances.

With this last sentence in mind, psychotherapy was initiated. Harry verbally poured out rage regarding his belief that he had been unjustly committed to the California Youth Authority. For three successive sessions he glared, ranted, and repeated over and over in the fashion of a cracked record, "Nine months for nothing! I didn't steal no car. I was just sittin' in it when they came and got me. I was just keepin' warm. Nine months for nothing!" This tirade against persecuting authority was for several days unaffected by the therapist's cautiously repeated reminder that, while he may have been unjustly accused of auto theft earlier, he had, by his own admission, just stolen two cars while escaping. "This," Harry roared, "was different. I *had* to take them cars because they were after me." Additionally, Harry accused numerous specific persons of persecuting him, and threatened great violence toward them.

In the fourth hour, Harry paused in his hate-ridden antiauthority filibuster long enough to mention that he liked to draw, specifically, to copy Walt Disney animals out of comic books. Partially in the hope of resting my weary ears, and partially to attempt an indirect penetration of Harry's verbal barricade of repetitive delusional phrases, I seized upon this opportunity to ask him to try some drawing then and there. He was at first frightened by the prospect of trying to draw without copying, and terrified of the subject matter which I asked him to produce—the human figure. He was, however, coaxed, encouraged, and applauded through the production of Drawing No. 1 before the hour was over. Drawings of the human figure often reflect inner conflicts of the artist.

For this drawing, and the ones produced in ten subsequent interviews, instructions were simple and relatively nonspecific. "Just draw a person. Try to do the best you can." In each session, when the drawing was completed, Harry was asked, "How do you feel about it? Are you satisfied with it? Is there anything you might feel like changing if you were doing it again?" He was given no suggestions or instructions in drawing technique. The drawings were done during the first quarter of each hour. The remaining portion was devoted to discussion of a variety of Harry's personal problems, which began to displace the "Nine months for nothing!" theme after the fourth interview.

A comparison of these drawings, in sequence, with the verbal content of the interviews which accompanied them no doubt brought smiles of great joy to Dr. S. Freud, if he were observing from somewhere in psychoanalysts' heaven. His concept of paranoid aggression as a reaction-formation[1] against repressed homosexual conflict appears to be illustrated convincingly in Harry's art. The course of verbal therapy during this period, extending from Drawing No. 1 through Drawing No. 11, may be divided roughly into four phases:

Phase (1). Harry's anguished, raging, expression of stereotyped, logic-tight, delusions of persecution (Drawings No. 1 and 2).

Phase (2). Harry's progressive use of the accepting relationship to permit himself to confide more and more of his underlying feelings. In the interview preceding Drawing No. 5 after struggling for some twenty minutes to gain courage, Harry repeated his fear that I would not like him if I knew "the truth." Then he confessed that he had run away from the institution to escape the pressure of stronger boys for sexual favors. He had semi-voluntarily performed fellatio on a few boys whose social acceptance he wanted to gain, and was then overwhelmed by demands and threats of beatings by many others who heard about it and desired similar services. Following Harry's catharsis, he seemed greatly relaxed. He was relieved to find that his therapist still accepted him as a person. Results of this session are quite evident in Drawing No. 5, where, for the first

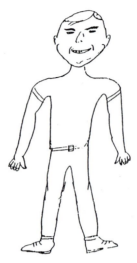

DRAWING NO. 1. Expressed dissatisfaction with legs and hands; redrew them and facial features. Still dissatisfied, but does not feel that he could improve on it.

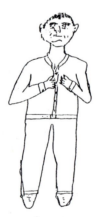

DRAWING NO. 2. Feels that the head is improved. Dislikes hands again — "too short." Redrew hands.

time, the facial expression becomes relaxed , smiling, and pleasant, as well as somewhat delicate and feminine.

Phase (3). Harry's expression of guilt feelings about his homosexual experiences, and his terrible fear that he might be "a queer."[1] I responded with supportive discussion of the psychosex-

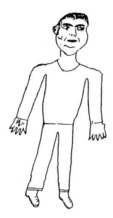

DRAWING NO. 3. Expressed lukewarm feeling of satisfaction. No changes. "Head looks better. Body is all right."

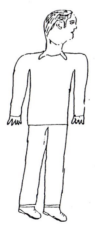

DRAWING NO. 4. Dissatisfied with hands once again. Redrew left one. Expressed moderate overall satisfaction, but ". . . not as good as last one."

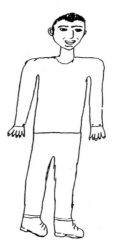

DRAWING NO. 5. "Looks better than any of the others." (How?) "The face looks more real."

ual plurality of all persons, and reassurance that there is nothing wrong with men having tender, passive components to their personalities — that this was perfectly normal, but that the important reality questions concerned one's choice of how these feelings are to be expressed. I asked whether or not Harry's homosexual acts had been effective in gaining for him the need satisfaction (social acceptance) which he sought.[2] Harry's progress in accepting his own feminine characteristics is reflected graphically in Drawings No. 5, 6, and 7.

Phase (4). Harry's assimilation of his new area of self-acceptance into a revised self-image. As he definitely chose to identify with masculinity, he systematically exchanged both the former pseudo-masculine, paranoid-aggressive features and the blatant feminine ones for an image of integrated broad-shouldered kindliness (Drawings No. 8 through 11). Harry's introduction of whiskers in Drawing No. 8, might suggest that he was using his therapist as an experimental ego-model during this phase of his search for a satisfying self-image, since the writer was at that time wearing a beard. While Drawing No. 11 still reveals some conflict and doubt, Harry expressed satisfaction with his product, and announced that he would not need to draw any more, but henceforth would prefer to devote all of the interview time to talking about himself, his problems, and his future. Harry no longer entertained the notion that he had been committed unjustly, and he was relating rationally and warmly to other staff members.

Verbal therapy, focused largely on reality factors — current problems in his relationships with peers and family was continued

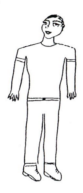

DRAWING NO. 6. (Smiling): "Head looks too much like a lady's." (Asked if that bothered him): "Yeah, I guess it does bother me some." (Asked if he would like to change anything about it): "No, I guess that's all right."

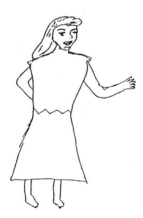

DRAWING NO. 7. (Started drawing face): "Guess I'll draw a girl this time. Is that O.K.?" Expressed satisfaction with results, except, ". . . not as good as if I took about an hour on it."

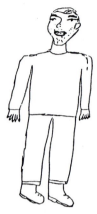

DRAWING NO. 8. Dissatisfied with left shoe: "Too big." Made minor erasure and change on shoe. Satisfied. No comment on whiskers.

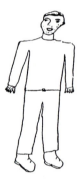

DRAWING NO. 9. "I'm so used to drawing them women now that the face looks like one. I have to put a beard on it to make it look like a man." (Apparently has been practicing alone in his spare time.)

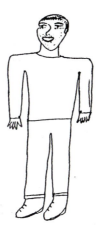

DRAWING NO. 10. "It's O.K." (Changes only left hand, adding fingernails.)

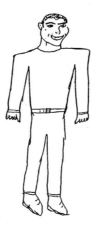

DRAWING NO. 11. "You put teeth in it, it doesn't look quite right either. Don't think I'll put 'em in." Explains that fingers are folded under, and that left ear can't be seen because head is turned. "I believe he's a better lookin' man. Don't think I'll need to draw any more of 'em."

weekly for twenty-eight more sessions. Harry was referred to parole, fairly well-liked by Escalon staff and peers, interested in finding a job, and looking forward to exploring an area in which he had never had any experience — dating girls.

SUMMARY

This case study has demonstrated the relationship between self-concept and the task of drawing the human figure. More specifically, it has graphically shown how the pseudomasculine, hyperaggressive defenses in an acute, if transient, paranoid reaction may serve as a mask for underlying problems of psychosexual identification. And it has shown one way in which an innovative adjunct can enhance the effects of verbal therapy.

NOTES

1. "Reaction-formation" means over-reacting to a threatening unconscious urge by exaggerated behavior in the opposite direction.
2. It is interesting that I unconsciously used this "Why Not? therapy" technique two years before I became aware of the concept and could consciously explain its value.

Chapter XI

Twister —
Brief Counseling Fails
to Change a Lifestyle

This case is included because it has always stuck in my craw as a therapeutic failure. My encounter with this young man took place very early in my Youth Authority career. I had not yet encountered the concepts, nor developed the techniques for "Why Not?" therapy. The traditional methods at my disposal at that time worked to establish rapport, but had no effect on Wayne Thompson's lifestyle.

The self-imposed nickname, "Twister," should have told me something. In the delinquentese of the day, "twist" meant to be caught, arrested, and sent off to do time. Wayne Thompson had selected a nickname to match his lifestyle. He had learned to cope inside correctional facilities where, off and on, he had spent eight of his seventeen years.

Twister knew how to "make it" with staff. As big bad "duke," he got no static from fellow inmates, and was employed as "monitor" by staff to maintain law and order in the ranks, which he did without having to lift a finger. An eyebrow was sufficient. He received special privileges and status from all sides. Although his world was small, in it he was a success.

By way of contrast, in his first nine years, and later, in intermittent excursions into the larger world outside the walls, he had been an abject failure. He had never achieved any status nor had any satisfying interpersonal relationships at any level of intimacy.

My first meeting with Twister occurred just after he had been referred by the Board for preparation of parole placement plans. He had been in the institution nine months for auto theft, and was due to be released the following month.

My notes on the six counseling sessions we held before his release follow. Unfortunately, I had not become acquainted with the "Why Not?" approach at that time or maybe I could have been of more help.

SESSION #1 NOTES

Wayne, or Twister, as he prefers to be called, referred himself to me. His problem, as presented, is that he isn't interested enough in staying outside an institution to "make it" when he is released next month. Additionally, he has a few new adventures he would like to try, just for a change of pace, such as ". . . armed robbery sounds like fun."

He described the high status he enjoys in the institution which he cannot achieve ". . . on the outs." Also, he suffers miserable relationships with his domineering mother and harsh, autocratic father.

Cars, he informed me, are tremendously important to him. That's why he has stolen five. Cars give him a feeling of bigness, of being ". . . one of the boys." His feelings about the armed robbery fantasy seem to stem from the same source — the desire to see himself as a "big man." (Which in turn implies that he is bothered by feelings that he is *not* a "big man.")

He said that he has been thinking about volunteering to extend his time in the institution in order to try to come to understand himself better before he leaves. (Really? I wonder if self-understanding is his motive, or if he is just looking for some way to avoid leaving this secure, satisfying little world for the frustrations and failures he always encounters on the outs.)

He does not appear to be a good candidate for personality counseling; but he is certainly not ready to succeed on parole. Therefore, I agreed to meet with him weekly until he leaves.

SESSION #2 NOTES

Twister had to be escorted to my office from "Seg" (segregation — the disciplinary lock up unit), where he had been placed after deliberately lighting up a smoke right in front of the group supervisor during a no smoking period. I inquired why he had done this. Twister responded with a detailed analysis of the supervisor he wanted to "shake up." He pictured the man as insecure, constantly afraid of losing control of the group, or individuals in it. This fearfulness, according to Twister, was obvious because of the supervisor's exaggerated attempts to overcontrol, his bossy style, complete inability to admit mistakes, and confusion in the face of any threat to his authority. Twister described the man also as a "scapegoater" who, when a boy quietly submits to his barking, applies more and more pressure and "controlling" measures until his victim breaks and becomes "insubordinate." If the "insubordination" is just the right amount, Twister explained, enough to frighten the man, but not enough to cause him to "write it up," it is the only way ". . . to get him off my back and quit messing over me." The man, he said, had been riding his back for a couple of days, and he enjoyed lighting the cigarette right in front of him just to watch him get confused and scared, not knowing quite how to handle it. The only trouble was that the man wrote him up and had him put in Seg — but, ". . . oh well, that's one of the risks of the game."

I commented that Twister's reaction to this man reminded me in some ways of his account last week of his relationship with his father.[1] He said, "Yeah. In a lot of ways he does remind me of my dad. I never thought of that before." I commented that he had been describing a lot of things that sounded like personal problems of the supervisor in question, and that apparently, he let this man's problems affect him to the point that he got himself in trouble. We developed this theme, drawing the parallel pattern of his relationship with his father — that often Twister got into trouble in response to autocratic, cold treatment by his father. He pondered this seriously, and said, "Hmmm." I said, "I wonder if you generally let your feelings about other people's behavior get you into trouble." Twister thought back about his numerous trips to Seg, and could recall only one that wasn't based on this pattern—not liking some-one's style and attempting to show him ". . . he's not such hot shit."

Twister boasted of his status among the boys, and the enjoyment he gets from being a "big wheel." I said, "Everyone likes to have some prestige, and you have found this is one way to get it." He replied, "I like it this way. It's the best. It makes me feel pretty good to hear some guy telling a new one, 'There's Twister Thomp-son. He's pretty bad, man.'" I asked, "In what other ways have you ever achieved any recognition?" He couldn't think of any. I said, "Well then, you really can't say this is the *best* way to get the feeling of being important because you have never achieved any-thing except in this area. You wouldn't know, for example, how it feels to have the general public look up to you for something you have accomplished. You get some recognition from being a big wheel with the boys all right, but it's from a very limited group of immature people. What is their recognition worth? Most other peo-ple would think it was kind of silly, and look down upon your status instead of up to it.[2] All you can really say is that this is the *only* way you have found to feel like somebody important, but not necessarily the *best* way, because you haven't experienced any others."

With this attempt to arouse some anxiety and dissatisfaction with his lifestyle, I closed the session.

SESSION #3 NOTES

Twister spent the entire hour talking about the great changes that have suddenly taken place in his attitude. He said that his ideas have jelled and everything that he has been mixed up about seems to be falling into place. I asked, "What do you suppose could account for this?" He explained that the Board's threat to send him to the Pres-ton School of Industry (a California Youth Authority Institution for older, more sophisticated delinquents) if he doesn't do an excellent program for the rest of his stay here shocked him into going to work on straightening out his thinking.

He reported becoming enraged at his father during a recent visit because his father refused to promise him permission to get a driv-er's license when he is paroled. Afterwards, Twister reported, he realized for the first time that his father has some reasons for denying him this privilege.

Many of his expressed values of last week were renounced in this session. For example, he pointed out the relative lack of value of his status in the firms (institutional power cliques) compared with acceptance and recognition in the outside world.

He described in detail the crusade he is undertaking to rid the institution of its social evils (many of which Twister perpetuated, if not instigated). He is breaking down the inmates segregation code, for example, and encouraging the different races to associate with each other. He is putting out the word to the firms to quit picking on "punks." In short, he is attempting to use his power to bring about a better society in his little world.

I complimented him on the mature thinking and actions, and added that a strong person can do a lot of good for people if he directs his strength into constructive channels. Twister said, "You know, I might like to be a supervisor some day."

SESSION #4 NOTES

Twister was depressed today, worrying about why the fine, mature attitudes expressed last time don't hold steady. He is plagued by recurring thoughts that he would *like* to go to Preston, that he will surely twist again within a few weeks of his release, and that he just doesn't care about anything.

I reflected* his gloomy feelings for most of the hour. He disclosed that his relationships with females, especially his mother, have been dismal. He contrasted this with the strong, positive relationship he has with another inmate named Wilson. Also, he pointed out that the loyalty and support given to a fellow by his "firm" is something worth treasuring. I said, "This is something most people get from their families. Right or wrong, succeed or fail, the family still loves you and stands ready to help." Twister said, "Hell! All my old lady ever says is that I have to stay locked

---

Rember, to "reflect" a feeling means to paraphrase it uncritically without agreeing or disagreeing. This communicates that the therapist is listening, cares, and understands.

up because I'm a menace to society." I reflected his feeling of bitterness about his mother's rejecting him, and he poured out a good deal more. When he had run down and sat mournfully staring at the floor, I said, "Nobody at home cared enough to sit down with you and try to understand how you feel, so you found Wilson to do it. Your family never gave you the secure feeling that they were behind you and rooting all the way, so you had to seek this loyalty from a firm in a correctional school." Twister pondered this in silence for a long time.

At last he asked, "Why is it my feelings don't stay the same? Always up and down. Last week I felt like doing a lot of good things. Then the least little thing makes me think I don't care at all and may as well mess up." In closing the hour, I tried to give him emotional support by answering, "Every kind of human growth works that way, Wayne. (He looked up and smiled when I called him by his real name.) It goes in ups and downs. When a baby is first learning to walk he looks pretty good for a few steps. Then, boom! Flat on his bottom. The next try he may not make it as far as he did the first time. But then look at him over a longer period of time. His ability to walk, on the whole, is improving, despite the ups and downs. That's the way it is with your ideas and attitudes — up and down, but gradually climbing and stabilizing. It can't happen all at once." He said, "I sure hope they get straightened out before I leave."

SESSION #5 NOTES

Anticipating his release in two weeks, Twister talked about the problems he will have to face when he goes home. His major concern was getting a driver's license, which his father says he can't have until after he has successfully completed his ninety day trial placement and is granted full parole status. Twister's view is that getting a license immediately and having legitimate access to a car would eliminate the temptation to steal a car when he has a long way to walk and sees one "waiting." I suggested that he discuss this with his parole officer as soon as he gets home, and maybe he will help persuade Wayne's father that the driver's license is a good idea. I asked what he thought would happen if his father proved unyielding. Twister thinks he can "sweat it" without getting into trouble. I said, "Ninety days isn't really forever."

Another worry was the fights Twister sees as inevitable when he hits the streets of his home neighborhood. He is in fact, caught between the need to protect his reputation as a "bad dude" and the probability of having his parole revoked if he fights. He noted that "on the outs" people don't realize how he feels when he wants to stay out of trouble, and think he is "chicken." I reflected his conflict, "You aren't really sure whether it's more important to stay out or to prevent people from thinking you are chicken." He concluded that maybe he could "let things slide" and not have to fight.

He spent the last few minutes describing his new job as "Seg Monitor," obviously enjoying his position of power over the other youths in the discipline unit, and exhibiting a remarkable identification with "the establishment" in this role.

SESSION #6 NOTES—FINAL

Twister immediately expressed his conviction that he will "get busted" again immediately following his release. Not only that, but he says he plans to do so. He wants to go to Preston to see if it is as tough as it is cracked up to be. He expressed a completely self-centered, immature set of values, denying any feelings for anyone or interest in the outside world. I said, "You are afraid there is no place for you in the outside world—afraid you will fail if you try to take responsibility for yourself." Twister denied this, insisting that he simply does not like to work because it is not pleasant, and that it is "pretty good" in institutions because ". . . you don't have to take people telling you what to do." He pointed out that if he were not satisfied with his job here, he could just cuss out the supervisor and get moved somewhere else, whereas he would starve with that kind of behavior on the outs. He added philosophically, "Why worry about things? Don't worry and you stay young." I asked, "But *how* young?" He winced a little, grasping my aspersion on his maturity. He continued expounding his abdication of responsibility for the rest of the hour. In closing our final interview, Twister thanked me for my "help." I wished him good luck and said, "I hope you find your place in the real world one of these days, Wayne, and learn how to be happy."

*****

Some three years later, a fellow staff member returned from a cross country vacation and told me, "I visited a number of institutions in the different states. Guess who I ran into in the Federal Reformatory in McAlester, Oklahoma! Twister Thompson! Transporting stolen cars across a state line."

Could I, with more time and better counseling techniques, have changed Twister Thompson, habitual prisoner, into Wayne Thompson, citizen? I'll never know. But it gnaws at me. "Why Not?" therapy might have turned the trick.

NOTES

1. It is interesting to speculate how much more effective it might have been to approach this theme from a need-analysis, "Why Not?" stance, instead of the traditional path I took.

2. If I had been skilled in "Why Not?" counseling at that time, I would have said something like, "You want other people to look up to you. Is there something wrong with that? No? Then let's look at your method of getting it. Is it really effective? Might there be better ways? What might they be?"

Chapter XII

Little Hitler —
Der Führer Loses Out
to a More Satisfying Ego Model

Robert Smally's delusional system was so rigid and bizarre that for the first eight weeks of therapy I aimed largely at establishing a warm relationship with him. This was successfully accomplished through sticking almost entirely to client-centered reflection techniques, punctuated by occasional questions aimed at stimulating him to test reality.

The supportive atmosphere of Escalon and my unswerving and uncritical personal acceptance of him, weird ideation and all, reduced his anxiety level to the point where he could accept gentle challenges to his delusional system. By our ninth session, Robert had related very positively to me. His thinking had become clear enough to permit me to switch to an emphasis on "Why Not?" therapy. From that point through the final ten sessions, his improvement was astonishing.

TO: Classification Committee
FROM: Clinical Psychologist
SUBJECT: SMALLY, Robert T.

This is a seriously disturbed boy who is resorting to a delusion system in order to cope with the frustrations of reality. He is well on his way to developing a paranoid schizophrenic psychosis. It is urgent that psychotherapeutic intervention be attempted immediately. Interviews are being scheduled. Immediate transfer to the Escalon program is recommended, where environmental stress will be reduced.

William B. Lewis
Clinical Psychologist II

It is interesting to note that throughout his nineteen weeks of individual treatment, Robert and I never once discussed his commitment offense, which was burglary. There are two reasons for this. One is that the fragile condition of his personality structure — on the verge of disintegrating into stark madness — seemed a much more crucial problem than his past delinquencies. The other is that Robert was also participating in small group counseling in the Escalon program, and was able to discuss his delinquencies in that setting.

SESSION #1 NOTES

This small, fifteen-year-old boy weaves a delusional tale which is both out of phase with reality and contradicted by his case file. Born in this country, but cast off early by his mother to be raised by an aunt and uncle after his father's death in an auto accident, Robert claims (and believes) that his father was a Major in the German Gestapo and his mother a Jewess who came to America before his birth. He also claims to have returned to Germany where, at age five, he lived for a year with his father. There, he says, he learned the true philosophy of the master race, which he now propounds vehemently, while intermittently cursing himself for having "half Jewish blood." I asked Robert if he has read *Mein Kampf*. He said, "Yes, a couple of years ago," and continued with his narration. He informed me that he had belonged to both a Youth Bund and a Communist Youth Group (at different times). He expressed hatred for the people in the world for mistreating him, and a wish to rise to a position of tremendous power, such as that enjoyed by Hitler, so he may avenge himself. He says he despises America and its philosophy of weakness. At another point he complained about not having freedom of speech.

Primarily concerned with establishing an accepting relationship,

I listened and noncritically reflected his thoughts and feelings throughout most of the hour. Toward the end, I did attempt to inject a bit of reality testing bait. I said that I was having trouble following his logic on one point. He had been speaking in favor of a hard, tough form of government, fascism, which is famous for not permitting freedom of speech, but then he complained about having his own speech curtailed. How come? He puzzled over this, but couldn't come up with an answer. I added, "Also, when you say the Arians are 'superior,' how do you mean that? Superior at what?" By superior, he explained, he meant more intelligent. He added that he always holds back on IQ tests because he doesn't want people to know he is bright. (Test results in his file indicate a dull-normal level of intelligence, but some of the concepts he handles in conversation make me think he is indeed much brighter than that, but is not functioning up to his potential due to his personality disturbance.)

SESSION #2 NOTES

Comparatively little of the fascistic ideological material emerged in today's session. Instead, Robert immediately focussed on the here and now, reporting how much more relaxed he feels since transferring into the Escalon program last week. He said it makes him feel peculiar for the supervisors to treat him in such a relaxed, kindly way. "Peculiar?" He clarified, "It always makes me suspicious when people act kind to me. I always think they are working an angle of some kind." I interpreted, "You are wondering if I am trying to trick you—if I am working an angle." He repeated that whenever adults treated him kindly in the past, they always had something up their sleeves. Then he proceeded to talk freely about himself for the rest of the hour. (Noncritically meeting his feelings of mistrust relieved them and opened the door for further communication.)

Robert touched on his feelings of loneliness and inadequacy. I resisted a temptation to relate these feelings to his grandiose, power-seeking fantasies, and continued to reflect his comments without interpretation or criticism. He mentioned the Arian superman doctrine again, this time, rather apologetically, in relation to his own brown hair and dark eyes. He hastened to explain that all Germans are not blue eyed blondes, although he admitted to being a little confused by Hitler's emphasis on the glories of this "ideal" complexion. I said that I sometimes wonder if Hitler's thinking might have been a little fuzzy — always making a big deal of his blond, blue eyed super race, while he, Goebles, Goering, and others among his top staff were, unexplainably, brunettes. Robert did not defend his hero's logic, saying, "I think I see what you mean."

In a giant step forward, Robert followed that concession with a statement that he, himself, always has a powerful need to "be right" in front of others, even when he doesn't know for sure that he is. He went on, without any assistance from me, to explain this, and his intellectual strivings, as products of his small stature and feelings of physical inadequacy. Again, I reflected his remarks without attempting to tamper with them.

SESSION #3 NOTES

Robert verbally attacked Mr. L., his trade supervisor, for most of the hour. The onslaught was strongly paranoid in flavor, accusing Mr. L. of having homosexual designs on Robert. He backed up the accusations with elaborate, pseudorealistic "examples" of behavior which "proved it."[1] Also, Robert reported, Mr. L. has started a rumor that he (Robert) is a homosexual, and that is why all the other boys stare at him now. I stuck with my relationship-building strategy, noncritically reflecting Robert's expressed ideas and feelings. He moved on to explore aloud his own conscious feelings and attitudes about homosexuality, which are characterized by fear and hostility.

Tiring of this theme, or perhaps feeling threatened by his own discussion of it, Robert switched to his old standby, praising Germany and criticizing the United States.

Our relationship has reached a point where I can intersperse a few provocative comments or questions among my reflections of his feelings, sometimes getting through his previously logic-tight delusional barrier, and eliciting some mild concessions to reality. For example, Robert was decrying American war movies which always show Germans surrendering, but never Americans. Instead of reflecting, "This seems unfair and prejudiced to you," I said, "That seems to be a pretty common human trait, wanting to look only at our good points – glorify ourselves – and show up the other fellow's bad points. I wonder how often the Germans like to show movies of Germans surrendering to Americans." Robert said, "I see what you mean."

SESSION #4 NOTES

Robert took off immediately on Germany, Hitler, war strategy, punishment of war criminals, and related subjects, propounding the Nazi viewpoint. I continued to listen, and reflect his feelings. Now, however, I can occasionally interpose a question or comment which points up possible inconsistencies in his thinking.

He asked if I thought he ought to become active in the Youth Bund again. I said that only he could make that decision about himself, but that it might be helpful to him to itemize some of the advantages and disadvantages of such a move. I asked him to think of as many pros and cons as he could, and I would write them down. Then he could take a look at them on paper and weigh them in trying to decide. Under advantages, Robert mentioned: (1) excitement, (2) feelings of importance, (3) social relationships within the group, (4) great opportunities for status and power if the group should "succeed," and (5) association with people whose ideas and values are similar to his own. As disadvantages, Robert listed: (1) obligations of membership might involve the commission of crimes and his being locked up again, (2) in the long run, mere *membership* would not satisfy his great desire for power and status, and (3) membership would limit his acceptance by larger society (which he says, sour grapes fashion, is of little importance to him, anyway.)

Robert abruptly abandoned this subject without announcing a decision. He turned to complaining about one of his living unit supervisors, Mr. S., for never giving him answers, but always putting him in a position where he has to think for himself. Robert doesn't like this because ". . . people have always told me what to do." I reflected, "You don't feel comfortable assuming responsibility for your own decisions like that." (Note: I had just done the same thing Mr. S. was being accused of – refusing to make Robert's decision about the Youth Bund for him, and his complaints about Mr. S. were probably actually aimed at me.) He agreed that this business of being forced to think for himself did make him uncomfortable.

Then, paradoxically, Robert spent the rest of the hour complaining about his aunt always trying to impose her will on him, refusing to recognize his views, opinions and desire to think independently and make his own decisions. I didn't point out the paradox, but encouraged the expression of his need for independence by reflecting, "You really want to think for yourself." He also expressed the feeling that his aunt treats her own son with favoritism, which makes Robert very hostile toward his cousin. He said that he gets along pretty well with his uncle, who advises him to ignore his aunt when she nags him. (It is interesting how he handled his conflict between wanting to have others think for him and at the same time resenting it when they do, by switching repeatedly back and forth between the two opposed positions, apparently without noticing the self-contradictions.) He closed the session expressing bitterness toward people who are always ". . . deciding what is best for me without even caring how *I* feel about it."

SESSION #5 NOTES

Robert devoted the entire hour to complaints and illustrations of being treated as a nonentity by his family. He said that they never consult him about his own feelings, wishes and thoughts on matters which concern him. I reflected all this material nonjudgmentally, offering only one interpretation at the end of the session. I said, "I wonder if all these experiences with people doing your thinking for you might have something to do with your desire to have great power and control over people—you know, like a Nazi leader."

SESSION #6 NOTES

Robert is relating very warmly to me at this point, relaxed and trusting. No political material surfaced at all today. Instead, Robert ventilated hostile feelings about Mr. G., on his living unit, who, Robert feels, dreams up fantastic ideas about what is going on in boys' minds. He resents Mr. G., telling him in a grandiose way that he can tell what Robert is planning, thinking or scheming, when, in fact, he is not planning, thinking or scheming anything. (Note: This is not all paranoid. Mr. G., does in fact have a bad habit of playing mental detective.) I continued with the client-centered style, listening, reflecting feelings, and accepting Robert's right to feel any way he wants.

He moved into an attack on himself, expressing disgust at his inability to face up to, and think through, his problems. He cited his tendency at home to escape to the drug store for a coke rather than work out problems which arose. Here, he escapes to his room and goes to sleep.

From this self-criticism, he sprang to another discussion of his family, this time expressing warm, positive feelings for them. He condemned himself for not having the drive and strength to make himself work, earn money, and do something nice for them. Instead, he said, they are always giving him whatever he wants in the way of material goods.

He complained about being forced to go to various institutional religious services, stating that he doesn't like to clutter up his mind with all that stuff, and that he has heard it all before. It bores him.

Then he switched to comparing California with "Back East" (Nebraska). He complained that the kids out here are different. They compete more, he said, to try to prove who is the toughest, who has the fastest or fanciest car, who is "coolest," and who can make the most broads. Those back East led simpler, less competitive lives, and enjoyed themselves in a more relaxed and wholesome way. His final point of comparison, incredible in the light of his earlier fascistic, superrace pronouncements, was the people back in Nebraska aren't as race prejudiced as they are here. I reflected, "It seems to you that California is worse than Back East when it comes to discriminating against minorities." Robert then, again incredibly, told me that people ought to treat each other fairly, and with respect, "live and let live," regardless of race. He even went so far as to say he wouldn't care if Negroes or Mexicans lived on the same street with him if they didn't let their houses get run down and shabby like some he has seen.

Robert told me, in closing, that these sessions with me really mean a lot to him, adding that he has never before in his life had a

chance to talk about his feelings to anyone ". . . who really understood."

SESSION #7 NOTES

Robert, articulately and with feeling, expressed his resentment of
the censorship in the institution which prevents him from keeping
up with current world events, and from reading literature on German political history. After reflecting his feelings on these matters
for some time, I began to pick up a personal slant in his remarks. I
asked, "Are you wondering how I stand on this? Whether I feel you
shouldn't read certain things?" He confessed that he has been wondering about this, because Mr. S., supervisor on the living unit has
told him he couldn't let Robert read certain articles without my
approval.

I said, "Okay. I'll tell you exactly where I stand. First, I am
subject to certain rules, just as everyone is, and I will not break
them, even though I don't always agree with them. If a school rule
applies to me, saying I must not allow you to do a certain thing, I
will not secretly allow you to do it. However, I do not believe in
censorship personally, and I am authorized to allow the boys I am
working with freedom of choice in their reading. The institution
does not give all staff, Mr. S., for example, this authority. I believe
that each person should be allowed to use his own intelligence, and
I do *not* believe in trying to force my ideas on you, or anyone. I may
tell you about them if you are interested, but you have the right to
decide for yourself what is right for you. I will not impose any
restrictions on your reading. In fact you are welcome to borrow any
of my books that interest you. On the other hand, it is not my responsibility to go out searching for books for you, and I will not
do it."

Robert expressed satisfaction with my position—that I am not
trying to rule his mind. He said that he had thought Mr. S., was
"doubletalking" him and "being sly" in telling him that he would
have to consult me on whether or not he could read certain articles,
but now he can see that Mr. S., was, in fact, being honest and
trying to avoid doing the wrong thing. I said, "Everyone has to

recognize the limits of his own authority." Robert sat in studious silence for several moments.

The last few minutes of the hour, Robert talked about problems of present day Germany, criticizing the United States for continuing to occupy West Germany. Instead of reflecting his feelings, I asked, "What do you suppose would happen if our troups just left there right now?" Robert discussed the possible reactions of the Russians to an American withdrawal, and thought they would try to invade and take over West Germany. At first he expressed confidence that the West Germans could resist such an invasion, then recalled the bloodshed and defeat of the Hungarians, and concluded, all through his own reasoning, that the question of American withdrawal is not as simple an issue as he thought at first. "Gee, I don't know."

SESSION #8 NOTES

In the past few weeks, Robert said, he has been becoming more and more aware of a desire to go home to his aunt and uncle. He expressed an intense and genuine wish to claim a place in the family. Almost poetically, he described a feeling that a fog has interfered with his view of life for the past couple of years, obscuring reality, and now it has dawned on him that he has been living an unreal, encapsulated life, divorcing himself from genuine human relationships. He expressed guilt about having been such a problem to his aunt and uncle, who tried so hard to reach him and give him love, which he rejected.

Robert cried bitter tears as he told me that his younger half-brother (who lives with Robert's mother and step-father), ". . . kind of likes to feel proud of me. He don't know that I ain't nothin' to be proud of." I met his feelings, "It really makes you sad to think that you haven't lived up to the little guy's image of you as a kind of hero." He said that he wanted to make it up to the people he has let down by ". . . being good and making them proud of me." He voiced a fear that he has invited complete rejection to the point where it may come about. A mixture of sadness and joy pervaded his thoughts about his aunt and uncle ". . . having to come clear up here to see me on Christmas."

Robert expressed great concern about "making classification," repeating his growing desire to go home and be part of his uncle and aunt's family. He wondered what I would say about him when the Institutional Classification Committee considers his readiness for parole. I reassured him that, the way things are going, I would not interfere with a referral to parole if the Committee feels his performance in other areas of his program warrants it. He was relieved, and said so.

I reminded him that he had mentioned "a few problems" he thought he should work on before leaving the institution, and asked him what they were. One of them, he said, was his inability to work well with, and take suggestions from, others. Another was inability to look people in the eye, a "shortcoming" often criticized by his uncle. I suggested that we discuss these next time.

SESSION #9 NOTES

Robert blasted the session open with the announcement that he is in the process of destroying all of his Nazi souvenirs, and that his whole way of looking at things has changed. He is not too clear on just what has taken place in his own thinking. He connects it all somehow with his recent recognition that he really wants people to like and accept him, rather than to have control over them. He said that the experience of being cared about, first by me, then other staff and wards, helped him to recognize his true need. Experiencing my unqualified acceptance of him as a person, distorted ideas and all, led him to realize that this, rather than Hitler-like power, is what he really wants out of life.

He said also that, though he is somewhat confused about what his mental state was and how it got that way, he has a feeling that he was seriously mentally sick, and getting worse, when he first met me. His former ideas about Nazis and superrace, he reported, now seem strange and unreal, ". . . almost as if it never happened." He is still interested in German History, but only as such. He no longer feels it is a part of him. He has just finished reading a book on the Mexican people, and was astonished to find himself as interested in it as he is in the German culture.

He expressed clearly his needs for love, acceptance and belongingness, and a feeling of confidence that he is worthy of these experiences and can achieve them now, since he has experienced them here. (I noted to myself, happily, that Robert's ego had begun to run on all cylinders, and guessed we could make use of this fact to bring about even more rapid progress through heavier emphasis on the ego-exercising "Why Not?" techniques.)

We took up one of the problems he mentioned at the close of our last session — Robert's wanting to work alone and free of other's suggestions and criticisms. I said, "You like to work independently and to avoid having others interfere with your ideas by suggesting things. Is there anything wrong with that?" Robert immediately accepted the fact that this need for independence is all right in itself, but added the observation that it could limit his opportunities for work in the future. I said, "Okay, there is nothing wrong with wanting to work independently, but you feel that insisting on this always, would interfere with getting something else you want — success on the job." He agreed, and said that he didn't think this would really pose a problem, because he can ". . . put up with people" and cooperate with them because he knows that this is what he must do to get what he wants.

Next, Robert said that he has a "religious problem." A bit of need exploration brought out that Robert really wants a satisfying religious belief, and that he has been pouting and rejecting a belief in God for several years because God didn't give him exactly what he asked for immediately. He said that he plans to approach religion again from his new way of looking at things — with an open mind — because he believes there is a lot in it for him which he refused to recognize in the past.

Robert said that he would like me to meet his family when they come up for a visit this weekend, but didn't see how this could be done, since I won't be working. I said that I would enjoy meeting them, and would be glad to do so in my home on Saturday if they wished to come by on their off-grounds visit. I said I would like to have Robert meet my family. He was elated, and fairly beamed as he assured me that his uncle and I would be great friends.

* * * * *

From this point onward, Robert's treatment was very much reality-oriented. In our ten remaining sessions, no further delusional material emerged. We clarified his needs through "Why Not?" procedures and discussed alternative methods of satisfying them in such areas as religion; his self-image and others' views of him with respect to intelligence; going to public school as opposed to a private "educational clinic" such as the one he attended earlier where he was frightened by the psychiatrist and his probing questions; his tendency to expect people to be like perfect parents — always caring, nurturing and reliable — and the fact that people can't really be counted on to fulfill this expectation; and guilt feelings regarding some transient homosexual fantasies, which Robert concluded probably wouldn't be a problem once he is free of the artificial, all male institutional environment.

Little Hitler went home as Robert, healthy American Boy.

NOTE

1. Such "examples," used to "prove" delusions, are common in paranoid conditions. They are referred to technically as "ideas or reference" and "logic-tight delusional barriers."

Chapter XIII

Silk Purse from a Sow's Ear: Client-Centered Approach Uncovers a Gem

Often I begin therapy using the "Client-Centered" or "Non-Directive" approach developed by Carl Rogers. I do this because I know of no better way to stimulate communication than listening and uncritically reflecting back the feelings expressed, showing that I understand and care about how the client feels, and that I respect his right to feel that way. This almost invariably frees the client of his fearful defensiveness and permits him to reveal quickly the areas which are troubling him.

As the problem patterns emerge, and the underlying legitimate needs begin to reveal themselves, I then may shift to a "Why Not?," analytic, or directive approach, and introduce appropriate auxilliary techniques such as art therapy, hypnotherapy, weight training with mirrors, or whatever best fits the individual's specific problem patterns and ability to communicate.

Sometimes, though, a client responds to client-centered reflection of his feelings in just the way Carl Rogers would say he should—pouring out his problems, clarifying his thinking about them, and coming up with his own solutions to them, with the therapist doing little beyond providing the accepting and noncritical atmosphere which permits the client to devote his energies to self-growth instead of self-defense. Such was the case with Lee Alberts. The results were astonishing. What at first appeared to be a real sow's ear personality turned into a silk purse, despite the old adage.

SESSION #1 NOTES

Lee is a 16-year-old whose most striking feature on first impression is abject crumbiness. He appears to have combed his hair with an eggbeater and from there down it gets worse. Staff have to force him to shower and change clothes.

His lengthy history of maladjustment is characterized more by parental neglect and rejection than by serious crimes. He fits well into the "cowed child" pattern. He has been involved, however, in hundreds of petty thefts over the years, and was committed to the Youth Authority for calling women, selected randomly from the phone book, and inviting them to have sex with him. (He found no takers.)

Though his emotional tone was flat and bland, he quickly related to me and spoke surprisingly freely in this first interview. After I told him that it was his hour and we could talk about anything he wanted to, he led off with a complaint that he doesn't know where to go when he eventually leaves the institution. I adopted a nondirective stance, and simply reflected his feelings. He said that he does not wish to return to his mother and stepfather. He and his stepfather were always at odds and seemed jealous of each other as competitors for mother's affections. He thinks he would like to live on a farm and work out of doors.

Lee pictured his mother as an unreliable, unstable, selfish person who has repeatedly disappointed him by failing to keep her many promises. She has often sloughed him onto various relatives, and disappeared. He described an incident as a small child when his mother left him with an aunt, supposedly for two days, and then went off with a boyfriend for an adventure in Palm Springs which, in fact, lasted for two weeks. She never writes to him. She has often taken off on vacations with different men, even after marrying his stepfather. He expressed sympathy for his stepfather, and commented that his mother shouldn't have got married if she wanted to keep running around with other men. If Lee ever marries, he said, it will be because he wants to be with his wife and family and do things with them. Lee agreed to continue meeting with me once a week.

SESSION #2 NOTES

Lee told me of a letter he has received from a couple at Edwards Air Force Base, offering to correspond with him regularly. They had met his tubercular stepfather and learned about Lee while on one of their regular visits to cheer up patients in the VA Hospital in San Fernando. Lee suggested that maybe he could go to live with these people. I reflected his feeling of longing for a stable and reliable home and family, but pointed out the reality that this couple are probably not looking for new family members, since they had only offered to write to him.

Lee again described his life of rejection and loneliness; feeling unwanted by anyone; and the competition with his stepfather for mother's love, which apparently was in short supply and dispensed freely to men outside the family circle.

SESSION #3 NOTES

Lee began by confessing that he habitually steals, and asked me why he does it and how to stop. One of his counselors on the living unit, said Lee, told him that the psychologist could solve this problem for him. I said, "That's not the way it works. I have no magic wand. All I can do is help you understand your problems a little more clearly so that *you* will be in a better position to solve them." I added that even if I could watch him all the time and keep him from stealing on the living unit, this would not be of much value when he leaves here and I am no longer with him.

Lee complained that he doesn't feel like a real person, but more like a robot, moving as if his impulses, or some other person, were pushing his buttons. He speculated that this passive, "nobody" self-image was probably a result of having been "blown around by the winds," dropped off at first one relative's home, then another, then a foster home, then an institution, without ever having any control over his own destiny or a feeling of belonging anywhere. I interspersed reflections such as, "You don't like being a robot . . . you are getting tired of having no control over your own life . . . you are beginning to think about taking responsibility for yourself." Lee reached the conclusion that he *must* assume the responsibility for supervising himself, or he will spend his life behind bars. He said that he has to do this right now, for he has been putting it off too long, and matters are getting worse all the time. I reflected these feelings, also.

Lee told me that he has surprised himself by learning things in the Escalon school program that he would have thought impossible. (He entered Escalon about three months ago. In the regular school program he had been placed in the class for the lowest academic group and was working with first grade books. At present he is progressing in high school general business and history. This remarkable improvement seems due largely to a changing self-image with increased self-esteem.) I reflected, "It makes you feel good to find out that you can do things you never thought you could do."

Lee again told me about his compulsive stealing and the guilt feelings that plague him after he steals. I told Lee, "A grown-up person has within himself a built in supervisor. This part of you has the job of controlling the little kid part of you that always wants to do things without caring whether it's good, bad, wise or foolish. Your inner supervisor seems to have been falling down on the job. It hides out when you need it, just before you steal, and then shows up to nag you about it when it's too late. Maybe you are going to have to kick your inner supervisor in the pants and make him stay on the job when you need him." Lee was amused by this schematization, and smiled weakly. He is still very flat emotionally.

SESSION #4 NOTES

Lee was in a little brighter, more cheerful mood than usual, and a little more emotional than I have seen him, although still on the bland side. He boasted that he has lost his "sticky fingers"—hasn't stolen anything since our session last week. I said, "You feel pretty good about being able to look yourself in the eye and say, 'I am not a thief. I used to be, but not any more.'" Lee affirmed that he does indeed feel good about it.

Lee described some new values he has discovered and adopted for himself, largely in the area of sensitivity to the feelings of other people, which he has lacked until now. He said that he has thought a lot about our last session, and has realized that he has always been concerned only for himself and his immediate wants; has never tried to meet anyone halfway, especially his stepfather; and has indeed been a robot, letting anyone who came along control him. He stated that he has definitely decided to do something about these things. As Lee phrased it, "God gave me a mind of my own, and I was supposed to use it; but I got into the habit of letting other people use it for me." He said that, looking back, he can see that he never gave his stepfather a chance to get along with him. He believes he can correct this now. Therefore, he has decided that he wants to return to his mother and stepfather, rather than go to a foster home.

Lee told me rather proudly that he has been giving cigarettes and candy to Paul, the cottage outcast, despite the risk of further rejection of himself by the rest of his peers. He delivered a surprisingly penetrating discourse on the values inherent in giving just to be giving, as opposed to trying to buy acceptance or some other favors. He described the warm feeling he derived from helping Paul to feel less lonely.

SESSION #5 NOTES

Lee's emotional flatness has disappeared. His speech was lively, warm and animated as he reported that his Senior Supervisor complimented him on his improved adjustment and rewarded him by moving him from the open dormitory into an honor room. (Ten of the fifty beds in the living unit are in private rooms.) I reflected his feelings of pride in this achievement.

He continued to talk about his newfound values, caring about others. His ideas show maturity, and involve sound human relations principles.

Lee told me how shocked he was when his mother, who had been dating a man whom Lee liked, showed up to visit him in Juvenile Hall with a different man whom Lee had never seen, and introduced him as her husband. Lee said that the angry, unhappy feelings caused by this experience probably doomed any chance for a good relationship between him and his stepfather. Lee said that he didn't want to get along with him, didn't try, and deliberately aimed at being hurtful and uncooperative. He now believes he can give the man a fair chance and get along with him.

He described a long series of runaways and placements in various facilities. His mother often deceived him. She took him to these facilities under false pretenses, then left him there. I chose to focus on the runaway pattern and commented that he seemed to have spent a lot of time trying to escape his problems by running away. He agreed, but added that this really didn't solve anything because most of his problems were in his own head. Consequently, they were still with him when he got to where he was going, as well as some new problems caused by the runaway itself. He added that he now sees that the runaway pattern just caused him more trouble, and he is going to stop it right now. He said that he is going to start facing his problems squarely and dealing with them, before he runs his way into San Quentin Prison.

Lee's continued productive response to a primarily client-centered approach is surprising me, since his initial appearance, bland, flat, and seemingly dull, gave me the false impression that not much could be accomplished with him beyond establishing a positive relationship.

Lee said that he would like to discontinue our meetings because he has "no more problems." I said that we can talk about this next time.

SESSION #6 NOTES

Lee said that he has changed his mind and would like to continue in therapy. He expressed concern about whether or not the staff will recommend him for parole. He has swung a bit too far, he feels, from passivity to assertiveness. (This is, in fact, great, but it scares him.) He has been getting into arguments with his Senior Supervisor because he has begun to speak out when he disagrees with some of his procedures (e.g., punishing the whole cottage population for the wrongdoings of one or two individuals.) Thus, he feels that he has lost favor with his Senior, and fears that this may cost him a recommendation for parole. He said, however, that he has very good relationships with the other staff.

Lee expressed unhappiness about receiving very little mail. His hospitalized stepfather writes about every two weeks. He hasn't heard from his mother for four months. I suggested that, realistically, if he expects to find any happiness in relationships with people, he may have to look to someone other than his mother. He agreed.

He again discussed possibilities for placement when he leaves the institution. At this point he favors placement on a farm or in a foster home.

SESSION #7 NOTES

Lee has been reading literature about becoming a Catholic Brother. He believes that the long school program would help to keep him out of trouble, as well as teach him ways to help people, which is the kind of work he would like to do. We discussed some of the pros and cons of such a plan. I suggested that he study it in greater detail with help from the Catholic Chaplain. I also pointed out that even if the Brotherhood program should not pan out, there are many other kinds of work which primarily aim to help other people. Lee said that his progress in school makes him believe that he can learn to succeed in one of the helping professions. He reminded me that before entering the Escalon specialized treatment program he had a second grade reading level, and now is passing in high school world history and business administration, as well as having turned in reports on twenty-three library books.[1] I asked how he accounted for this extremely rapid improvement. He said, "I guess I didn't have any self-confidence before." I reflected and clarified, "You have changed your thinking about yourself. Before, you couldn't do it just because you believed you couldn't do it. That sort of paralyzed you." He said, "Yeah. That's right. I was sure I couldn't do it, so I didn't even try. And, you know, I think that is true in other ways, too. I think I could have worked out getting along with my stepfather, but I didn't believe I could, so I didn't try." I said, profoundly, "Mmm hmm." (Give this kid an accepting atmosphere, and he does his own therapy.)

SESSION #8 NOTES

Lee asked if I thought he has "improved enough" to be recommended for parole when the Classification Committee reviews his case next week. I did not offer the reassurance he was seeking, but, rather, reflected, "You are concerned about how I see you at this point." Then I turned the question back to him. (Working on his own self-concept is much more valuable to him than any reassuring words from me could be.) I asked, "Lee, how do you see yourself in this regard?" He responded with a number of improvements he sees in himself. Among them were greater ability to accept disappointments without withdrawing into a shell or blowing up; self-confidence; ability to see through, and resist, peers' attempts to agitate and manipulate him; clearer thinking; and a growing ability to think of effective ways to solve problems which arise from day to day. He illustrated each of those areas with specific examples.

We closed the hour on the subject of effective problem solving, defining it as, "Something you can do that will get you what you want without creating new problems as bad (or worse) than the one you started with."

SESSION #9 NOTES

Lee first expressed "nervousness" about his Classification Committee review, which takes place tomorrow. Then he continued with last week's theme, describing and illustrating positive changes that he sees in himself. These included improved ability to grasp and use social values—to understand what is going on in the social interactions he observes around him or participates in. He also believes that he looks better than he did because he is taking better care of himself. (His new interest in personal hygiene became apparent in our fourth session. Since then he has been keeping clean, dressing neatly, and combing his hair, without being prodded by staff, according to the reports.)

He commented that a few months ago he didn't particularly care whether he went home or stayed in the institution, but now it has become very important to him. I asked, "Why?" Lee explained that he sees things much differently now than he did before. "For example," he said, "I can see now that laws are made to help people live together and get along. I used to think they were just to try to keep me from doing anything, and didn't have any other purpose."

Lee elaborated on a number of his new concepts, attitudes and feelings. He closed by stating that it is interesting to understand all of these "new ideas," but he thinks that what he needs now is a chance to try them out in the real world. That is why he really wants to go home.

CONCLUSION

Lee was recommended for parole. We met six more times, reviewing, tapering off, gradually switching to a social conversation mode, preparing Lee for the termination of our relationship. To the end, his response to client-centered reflection was so rich and growth oriented that adding other techniques would have been superfluous.

When this young man came to the institution his self-esteem was all but nonexistent. He had but the foggiest notion of who he was at any level of interpersonal intimacy. Almost all of his relationships in the past, one-to-one, small group, and larger group, had been meager and unsatisfying. They failed to give him a sound sense of identity. Consequently, he soaked up every aspect of the treatment program to which he was exposed. He discovered who he is at a one-to-one level in therapy. He added several other dimensions through relationships in the treatment-oriented classroom, the Escalon living unit *milieu*, small group counseling, and as a participant in the large, cottage community meetings, which concern themselves with problems in everyday living as members of a community. His personality growth far exceeded my expectations.

Lee had to return, upon his release, to the same old emotionally impoverished, chaotic family situation that sent him here in the first place. However, I believe that he went home armed with new inner strength which will give him a fighting chance to cope with it. He knows now that positive interpersonal experiences are possible. He will seek, and find them.

NOTE

1. This dramatic improvement may sound impossible, but, in fact, over the years I have worked with several young people who suddenly jumped from non-reader to high school level scores in the course of brief therapy. They had already absorbed the know-how, but psychological blocks prevented them from being able to use it.

Chapter XIV

If It Ain't Broke, Don't Fix It: Suicidal Obsession Erased in Four Sessions

Not everyone who seeks individual therapy wants, or needs, a complete personality overhaul. When your car's spark plugs need changing, you don't normally ask the mechanic to rebuild the whole engine.

So it was with Jake Best, age 17, depressed and obsessed with suicidal thoughts. Otherwise, Jake's self-image at a one-to-one level of intimacy was pretty sound. He had close friends, and dated girls before coming to the institution for "joy riding" (unauthorized car "borrowing"). He just didn't show any need for intensive, long-term, one-to-one therapy.

Jake did lack a sound self-concept at the level of small group interaction, and at the less intimate level of responsible membership in a community. He had been filling some ego gaps at these levels for several months through small group counseling, the Escalon social environment, and the large group community meetings when he asked to see me privately because he couldn't shed a preoccupation with suicide.

There are many forms of depression, many degrees of severity, and many causes. For example, simple reaction to a loss of a loved one; biochemical malfunction; genetic predisposition; and unconscious misdirection of hostility. Consequently, appropriate treatments range from simple supportive counseling through insight therapy, chemicals and electroshock. Each of these has its place, depending upon causative factors in each case.

The depression we are concerned with in Jake's case is the kind which results from displacing hostility inward, onto the self. The way this works is that someone does something to frustrate, hurt and anger the victim. The perpetrator is a powerful figure in the victim's world (e.g., an employer, a mother, a college professor who could flunk one out of school). It is too dangerous to express anger directly toward this menacing person, but it does not just evaporate. Anger may hide, or disguise itself, but it is still there, seeking an outlet until it finds one.

One common way to deal with this kind of anger is to take it out on a target safer than the one who caused it. The boss humiliates us by chewing us out in front of coworkers. We forget it (consciously) over a couple of beers on the way home, and then kick the dog off the porch, spank the kids for making so much noise, and ask the wife why the hell she never has dinner ready when we get home.

If one does not wish to displace his anger onto innocent bystanders, there is yet another alternative. One can swallow the anger—turn it inward onto the self. In this form, the anger is experienced as depression. The victim feels low, rotten, and hopeless and doesn't know why. He feels like kicking *himself* off of the porch, or worse, off of a chair with a rope around his neck. Worse yet, he sometimes does it.

Often an intervention is vitally important, yet may not be very difficult or time consuming. Such was the case with Jake.

SESSION #1 NOTES

Jake said that he requested to see me because he has recurring thoughts about killing himself. One of his counselors suggested that I might be able to help. His demeanor was very low key; his speech slow and effortful. Depression was apparent. I said, "You are really feeling down in the dumps."[1] Jake began telling me how low he did feel. As I reflected his feelings, he spent half of the hour telling me how miserable he was, and how hopeless everything seemed to him. He cried.

After airing his depressed feelings, Jake began to elaborate on the suicidal thoughts that have been plaguing him for several months. The thought of killing himself comes to him over and over throughout the day, frightening and confusing him. He said, "I get the

feeling of not knowing what I am doing when I think about that."
He went on to say that sometimes he is afraid that he might really do
it. In fact, he confided at last, he did try it once. The car that he
stole for "joyriding" was in fact stolen for the purpose of killing
himself. He crashed it in a ditch trying to die. He did not tell this to
the police.

Toward the end of the hour Jake introduced a new theme, severe
rejection and "hate" by his father. He described his father's domineering behavior, constant criticism, and innumerable beatings
administered. (Note: Possible source of Jake's "anger-turned-
inward" depression.) Jake reported all of this mechanically, almost
in a monotone, showing no emotion.

I invited Jake to meet with me once a week for a while so we can
discuss these things further, and maybe get a little better understanding of his suicidal preoccupation.

I alerted living unit staff to keep a careful, but informal, watch on
Jake, just in case. The interest he showed in continuing our discussion suggests that a suicide attempt is not probable right now, but
neither is it out of the question.

SESSION #2 NOTES

After a slow, stumbling start, Jake's speech gradually warmed up
and became quicker and more spontaneous than it has been so far.

Jake told me about an attempt to run away with his girlfriend,
also 17, which failed, and led to her current residency in Juvenile
Hall. Jake, employed full-time, had, in gentlemanly fashion, asked
the girl's father for permission to marry her. The father, however,
declined to grant his blessings. Instead, he called Jake a sonofabitch
and threatened to cut his throat. Subsequently, when their attempt
to elope failed and his girl wound up in the pokey, it occurred to
Jake that the only reasonable thing to do would be to steal a car and
commit suicide in it. (Jake had his own car once, but, while he was
in Juvenile Hall, his father sold it and kept the money.)

I suggested to Jake that if he and his girl can have a little pa-
tience, she will soon reach the legal age of consent, and if they still
want to marry, they can, with or without her father's blessings. Jake
said, "Hey! I never thought of that."

For the remainder of the hour, Jake returned to the theme of his horrible relationship with his own father. Jake flunked out of school for falling asleep in class every day. His father, he said, got drunk every night, then woke Jake up and forced him to drive him around all night to bars and liquor stores. The only place Jake could get any sleep was in school.

For one brief period Jake and his father became allies against a common foe, a man with whom Jake's mother was having an affair. After a few months, however, the friendliness between Jake and his father subsided and the relationship returned to its norm — hateful, bitter, sick.

Although, Jake says, his father treats him fairly decently when he comes to visit, they just do not talk about anything important. It is a kind of non-relationship — just going through the motions. Jake said that maybe his best chance for "making it" on parole would be to live with one of several uncles in Oklahoma.

SESSION #3 NOTES

Jake opened with a comment that his suicidal thoughts are not bothering him much now. They cross his mind only once in a while, and quickly vanish.

Beyond that, the entire hour was devoted to a highly angry, bitter outpouring of his feelings toward his father. No mechanical, depressed monotone this time. Jake was raging, and he raged and he raged! He raged about mental oppression, lack of trust, arbitrary demands, stealing his car, and making him flunk out of school, not to mention the years of brutal physical beatings. At the end of the hour, Jake just sighed, and kind of ran out of gas.

I was able to point out to Jake (for the first time using a "Why Not?" therapy technique) that through all of the thunder and lightning that he let fly, he was really expressing a need to be independent — to think his own thoughts and make his own decisions without somebody else telling him how, or criticizing him. Jake pondered this, and then agreed enthusiastically that this is indeed what he wants. I cleared the legitimacy of this need with his ego, "Is there something the matter with that — wanting to be able to think for yourself and make your own decisions without being attacked and criticized?" He said, "No way! I have a right to want that." I said, "Great! Now, all you have to do is look at the ways you have been trying to accomplish this. Running away with your girl? Crashing the car? Did these get you the independence that you want? If these haven't been working, maybe we need to try to think of what *will* work. Well, we're out of time. See you next week."

SESSION #4 NOTES

Jake told me that he has given a lot of thought to what we discussed last week — approaches he might take to achieving the independence that he wants. Although he did not really think about it before, he said, he has suddenly realized that he, as well as his girlfriend, will soon reach the legal age of consent. This, plus recent positive changes he believes he has detected in his parents' attitude, make him think that he has a pretty good chance of getting along with them until he gets another job, turns eighteen, and can move out on his own. He believes that this alternative would be more effective in achieving independence than going to Oklahoma to live with his uncles, primarily because the job market in California is better. Should life with his parents again prove unbearable, he will ask his parole agent to assist him in moving to Oklahoma. If he cannot find a job in Oklahoma, he plans to join the armed forces and learn the mechanics trade, which he wishes to pursue as a career. He really has done some thoughtful planning, and has pretty well covered all the bases.

Jake briefly discussed the suicidal thoughts that brought him to see me in the first place. They have disappeared entirely. Jake said that they prevented him from making any plans for the future, because he had been so preoccupied and confused by them. I asked what he thought had caused them. He was able to relate them to feeling trapped in dependency on his abusive father, and being unable to see any way out.

I pointed out to Jake in a summarizing interpretation that sometimes when we are angry and cannot express it or do anything about it, we may just swallow it, getting angry at ourselves, depressed, and having self-destructive thoughts. Jake said that getting the anger toward his father out in the open and off his chest had been very helpful. He has had no suicidal thoughts since that session.

Jake again commented that he seems to have his problems straightened out now. I said, "Then maybe we don't need to continue our talks." He agreed. I said, "Well, why don't we stop them? We can leave it this way. If anything comes up that you do want to talk over with me, drop me a note and we can get together." Jake said that that sounded like a good plan, thanked me for my help, and took his leave.

CONCLUSION

Once again, client-centered technique at first encouraged Jake to ventilate his feelings of depression and identify his rage. This then permitted me to intervene with "Why Not?" therapy for the "mop up" (problem resolution, development of options and reframing Jake's legitimate need to be independent).

Jake never requested another interview in his remaining months in the institution. Reports on his progress in other areas of the program continued to be good. In a few informal encounters, just in passing, he seemed happy, talkative and self-assured. He said that his suicidal ideas had never returned.

I could have probed and dug up other things to talk about, extending the one-to-one therapy. But why? Jake got what he came for in four sessions. If it ain't broke, don't fix it.

NOTE

1. This technique, called "meeting one's feelings," is very useful in encouraging emotionally upset people to ventilate their feelings and explore why they are upset. The process often calms them.

Chapter XV

President of the Firm: Murder in the Making

One disadvantage of trying to do therapy in a correctional facility is that sometimes the bureaucracy won't permit it. Of course I can't be sure that the end result would have been different if the Classification Committee had let me continue to work with Buck Douglas. But they didn't. They transferred him to another institution for disciplinary reasons. I will always wonder if his continuation in therapy would have prevented what eventually happened.

In late 1957, when Buck Douglas was seventeen and first came to me for therapy, the Paso Robles institution was known throughout the Youth Authority for its unique informal social structure, the "firm" system. I was never able to learn where the term, "firm" originated. Apparently the system "just grew" like Topsy, without official sanction, almost from when the institution opened in 1948. "Old timer staff" could not remember when the firms did not exist.[1]

In this social hierarchy the residents divided themselves into five classes. The self-proclaimed coolest, toughest Whites called themselves the "Straight Firm." Ranking alongside the "Straights" were the "Bloods" (nowadays called Blacks) and the "Mexicans" (now called Chicanos). Whites who had some social standing, but were not cool enough to be accepted by the Straights, formed the largest firm, and called themselves the "Semi-straights." The unfortunate souls who were not acceptable to any of the four firms formed the fifth, and lowest stratum of the society. Although they had no organization, they were referred to, individually and collectively, as the "Punks." The Punks were mostly Whites because the Blacks accounted for only twenty-nine, and the Chicanos a mere seventeen percent of the overall population. These two minority firms needed all the manpower they could get in order to keep their military strength on a par with the Straights.[2] Punks were usually cowed child syndrome types who were afraid to fight, and who yielded their meager possessions, cigarettes, candy, or even their bodies[3] upon demand by their "superiors."

The reason I explain all of this is that Buck Douglas, the subject of this chapter was very big on firms. His uppermost concern was his status in the eyes of his peers.

SESSION #1 NOTES

Buck is a physically well developed young man who enjoys a reputation as a fearless fighter, and is currently the "president" of the Straight Firm in his living unit. He was recently placed in the Escalon program at his own request because his fighting was getting him into trouble so often that he feared he was never going to "make the program" and earn a referral to parole. Unfortunately, his aggressive behavior toward weaker boys was so disruptive that Buck got himself kicked out of Escalon and into the Potrero disciplinary unit within two days.[4]

Buck refused to return to a regular cottage program without seeing me to find out why he was expelled from Escalon before he had a chance to solve his fighting problem. I was the one who agreed to give him a trial in Escalon (against my better judgment).

When Buck arrived, demanding an explanation, I gave him one. I explained that one purpose of Escalon was to provide a secure atmosphere for its wards where, free from fear, they could concentrate on understanding themselves and working through their problems. He came into their program like hell on wheels, trying to "shape up" this group of "Punks" by hitting them, pressuring them for their goodies, and trying to make it clear that he was a superior being to whom they should kowtow. The other wards did not agree with his evaluation of himself, and neither did living unit staff, and neither did I, so we all agreed to kick him out so he couldn't continue to ruin the program for everybody else.

To my surprise, Buck accepted this confrontation without a rebuttal, and asked me if I would see him regularly to discuss his problems, if he went back to a regular cottage program. Despite my reservations about the amenability to treatment of Buck's severe character disorder, I agreed to see him weekly because of his actively requesting treatment.

I said, "Okay, Buck. We've got a deal. This is our first session. What do you want to talk about?"

Buck began by telling me that his mother had written to him recently announcing that she did not want him at home anymore, and that he would have to be paroled to a foster home. As I reflected his feelings, their intensity increased. He poured out bitter hurt and anger toward his mother for rejecting him.

He then generalized his angry feelings to include all people in authority, and "especially to Punks." (Safe targets for his displaced hostility.) As I reflected these feelings, he began to link them with homicidal fantasies. He said he often thinks, and dreams, about killing someone.

In the final portion of the hour, Buck brought forth the fear that his terrible anger may eventually destroy him. I gave him some reassurance that such does not have to be the case. As he gradually begins to understand his feelings more and more, I told him, he will become aware that there is a big difference between *having* a feeling and acting it out.

SESSION #2 NOTES

Buck returned to a regular cottage, lasted two days, and is now back in Potrero for fighting. He has been so unruly and hostile that Potrero staff feared to send him to my office, even under escort, so I went down there and held our session in Buck's lock-up room.

Buck blew off steam for the whole hour about being persecuted by people in general, and staff in particular. He attributed all his difficulties to external forces—people who are "messing over"[5] him. I simply reflected these feelings, encouraging their ventilation, but neither disagreeing with them, nor reinforcing them by agreeing with them.

SESSION #3 NOTES

Buck is again back in a regular cottage program.

Subject matter of today's session at first centered on cottage activities and relationships, and Buck's feelings about them. He complained at length about the new assigned seating program (aimed at preventing firm members from sitting together and hatching a "rat pack" or some other skullduggery). Buck opined that it is unfair and degrading to make "people" sit between Punks and Bloods and Mexicans. (This elitist frame of reference of Buck's is so ingrained and real to him that I wonder if I'll ever be able to make a dent in it.)

The theme returned to Buck's hostility and his fear that it will eventually cause his own destruction. He described some of his homicidal dreams. One in particular has been recurring almost nightly for several weeks. It frightens him because it is so real. In it, Buck repeatedly stabs a particular boy (the same one each time) with a knife while accomplices (also the same each time) hold him down. Buck described the victim as having ". . . very smooth skin — almost too smooth — like a girl's." I asked if the girl-like skin might have something to do with his feelings about the boy, or his stabbing. Buck quickly denied any such relationship, but then went on to say that he had "made out" with a few boys since coming to the institution eleven months ago. He suddenly blushed and began to stammer, as if he realized that he had confided more than he wanted to. He defensively explained that such behavior is the custom here, that everyone does it from time to time, that it is all in fun, that he never even thought about carrying it beyond kissing, and that he had only done it with a few guys that he "really liked — you know, really straight guys, not sex punks or anything like that." I asked if he ever thought about making out with the smooth-skinned guy that he stabbed in his dreams. Buck hotly denied this on the grounds that the one in the dream is a punk, and he would never make out with punks.

It seems probable to me at this point that much of Buck's aggressive, hypermasculine behavior is a defense against his own homosexual impulses threatening to break into consciousness — the classical dynamics behind many paranoid reactions. This, coupled with the homicidal fantasies and dreams, suggests that unless therapeutic intervention is successful, Buck could in fact develop a homicidal paranoid reaction and attempt to kill someone — a "punk" *or* an authority figure under certain circumstances.

Buck immediately jumped away from this threatening topic, sex with a punk, and returned to a discussion of the assigned seating program. His ideas were confused. He alternately talked about not believing in discrimination because of race or weakness and proclaimed his own superior status as a "straight stud" who should not be forced to sit next to those Bloods and Punks. (Hopefully, I will be able to help him become aware of his self-contradictions and use of logic-tight compartmentalization[6] if our relationship eventually becomes strong enough to permit such interpretations.)

Buck mentioned nonchalantly that his mother has decided to take him back after all. She has moved to this city to await his parole. Emotionally, it seemed as if he couldn't care less.

SESSION #4 NOTES

We have learned that Buck's mother was hospitalized locally, reason unknown, and then transferred to Camarillo, a state mental hospital. Buck wondered if a furlough to visit her might be arranged. I told him that it would not be possible to furlough him in her care while she herself was under hospital care. He accepted this without comment.

Buck launched a discussion of his feelings about race relations. He told me that it really upsets him and makes him angry to see White girls associating with Negro males. For some time he blew off outraged feelings on this issue. I ventured the interpretation that there seemed to be an element of jealousy in what he was saying. I asked, "Do you fear that those girls might be comparing you with the Negroes as lovers?" This question made Buck very uncomfortable. He stammered, "Well, they always say that Bloods have big cocks." I said, "It bothers you that the girls might like them better than you." Buck changed the subject.

He boasted about his prowess as a fighter, and about not being scared of anybody (obviously as a defense against the near exposure of his sexual inadequacy feelings). Eventually, I asked Buck if he had any idea why willingness to fight, and not being chicken was so important to him, pointing out that millions of people wouldn't think that is important at all. Instead, they judge people's worth on such things as honesty, kindness, ability to work, sense of humor, and how they treat other people. Buck could not grasp the concept, or at least could not formulate an answer.

SESSION #5 NOTES

Buck began by boasting about his progress at conforming to program rules, and at controlling his temper. He hasn't been in a fight all week, and has been appointed as one of the two monitors[7] for the cottage.

A problem has developed as a result of Buck's having been appointed to the "have muscles, will travel" position. The other monitor is a Mexican, and the one whom Buck replaced was a Blood (graduated to parole).

Buck said that the Bloods resent him in the job, and want to have him replaced by another of their own. Consequently, they resist his leadership in every way possible. Buck said that, in his view, every person should be treated the same regardless of skin color. (He added that his thinking along these lines has come about just since our last meeting.) I told Buck that I could think of two possible approaches he might take to this problem. One is to tell the group his belief in racial impartiality, assure them that he will be fair, and ask for their cooperation. The other is to talk to staff and suggest that a third monitor (Negro) be added to the system, so that all three of the recognized ethnic groups will feel represented.

SESSION #6 NOTES

The Classification Committee[8] has informed Buck that his recent progress (conforming to rules) has earned him their consideration for a recommendation for parole,[9] providing that I approved from a clinical standpoint. Buck asked me if I would recommend him for parole at present. (I wouldn't because I think he is dangerous, and I don't think that he believes he is ready.) I asked "How do you feel about it yourself?" He said, "In a way I want to get out, but in a way I don't." "How is that?," I asked. Buck discussed at some length the feelings of security afforded him by the structured institutional environment. He expressed fear of facing an unknown family in a foster home placement while awaiting his mother's release from the mental hospital.

Buck devoted the remainder of the hour to the expression of hostility toward his stepfather. He recited a number of incidents (true, or paranoid distortions, I don't know) in which his stepfather deliberately set him up to get in trouble, and others in which he went out of his way to destroy Buck's friendships and romantic relationships. He explained that his stepfather hates him because he (Buck) looks like his natural father.

Buck's final remark was that he has changed his thinking about staff "messing over boys." He no longer believes this to be true. He now says that he was just "thinking that" in order to justify his own unacceptable behavior.

Buck is really ambivalent about wanting to be paroled. He is attempting to manipulate me, alternately, into squelching his referral to parole for clinical reasons, and endorsing it because he has become such a wholesome, clear-thinking, good citizen.

SESSION #7 NOTES

Buck came in today complaining about not being able to remember "anything." I asked, "What do you mean?" He described in great detail a number of incidents which he "could not remember." I asked, "How are you able to tell me about these things if you can't remember them?" He said that his friends told him about them. I said, "I wonder how you can remember what your friends told you. Your memory seems to be working fine there." He said, "I don't know." (Has he truly experienced amnesia for some of his behavioral episodes, or is this another attempt to impress me that he is not well enough to be referred to parole? I don't know.) I asked him if he thinks this memory problem is severe enough to keep him from "making it" on parole. His pendulum swung again, and he assured me that these memory lapses should not be permitted to prevent his referral. "I probably can't remember things because I've been here too long."

I encouraged Buck to explore his feelings about his mother's "breakdown." (We have learned that she is suffering an acute psychotic episode.) He could not articulate his feelings very well, but enough emerged to permit me to point out that he seemed afraid that the same thing could happen to him. He did not respond, but appeared to be very uncomfortable.

SESSION #8 NOTES

Buck reported that his memory problem has completely cleared up since last week. He can remember everything just fine now. I confronted him, "Buck, you never did have a memory problem. You were just trying to con me, although I'm not sure into what. I think you try to con people a lot." At first he denied this, saying that, though capable of conning, he never does it. I confronted him with several examples of his attempts to manipulate me. Eventually he gave up and admitted that he does enjoy manipulating people. We discussed various kinds of conning that people do, ranging from bunco artists through crooked salesmen, politicians, honest salesmen, teachers trying to persuade students to learn, to the ordinary guy on the street trying to bargain for something he wants. Buck said that he believes only in "honest conning"—the kind that doesn't hurt anybody. I said, "I think you believe in whatever kind of conning that will be to your advantage."[10]

SESSION #9 NOTES

Buck spent the whole hour describing his interpersonal woes in school. The Bloods in his classroom have hinted that they are planning to rat pack him because of the resentment of him as a monitor on his cottage. The "Straights" in the class are mostly from other living units. They have told Buck that they will not "jump for him" (fight) if the Bloods do rat pack him. They say the reason is that he has turned chicken and doesn't fight any more. Buck has a dilemma. He doesn't want to jeopardize his possible referral to parole by fighting, yet he feels a strong need to ". . . straighten out them dudes by kicking some ass." I suggested that in our next session maybe we should look into the process by which he has managed to make enemies of the Bloods *and* the Straights in his class.

SESSION #10 NOTES

Buck is back in Potrero, this time for planning an escape. Staff discovered his window bars sawed, and the gear he was planning to take with him stashed under the bed. They snatched him out of class and hauled him away to lock-up.

Buck said that he thinks the Classification Committee may ask the Board to transfer him to Preston School of Industry, which houses older, more criminally sophisticated wards. I told him that I thought the best thing for him would be to stay here and continue in therapy. I also told him that my report to the Classification Committee would not have endorsed a referral to parole at this time because I don't think he is ready to succeed on parole. Anyway, his escape attempt has eliminated any positive consideration the Committee might have given him as a candidate for parole. He said that he would like to stay here and continue in therapy, rather than go to Preston. I assured him that I would recommend that alternative in my clinical report to the Committee, but added that he should not set his hopes too high because the Committee is not obligated to follow my recommendation.

CONCLUSION

I submitted my clinical evaluation of Buck to the Classification Committee. In it I stressed Buck's confusion and anxiety about his sexuality, and discussed the homicidal fantasies and dreams generated by these conflicts. I pointed out that unless these problems could be resolved through continued therapy, Buck would have a high potential for actually attempting murder on someone in the future. I recommended to the Committee that Buck not be transferred so that I could continue to work with him in an attempt to defuse the bomb he was carrying around in his head. I stated that reducing his potential for murder was much more important than punishing him for his escape attempt.

The Classification Committee transferred Buck to Preston. I never saw him again.

Some twenty years later I recognized Buck, then in his mid-thirties, on a "wanted" poster in an adult parole office.

Armed with a revolver, on a lonely road, Buck and an accomplice had intercepted two prison guards who were transporting a convict to court. In the process of carrying out the planned escape, the accomplice held one of the guards down while, at point-blank range, Buck blew him away.

NOTES

1. Seven years later, when all living unit programs had been restructured as therapeutic communities, with staff trained to provide individual, small group and large group counseling to all residents, the firms miraculously evaporated. They just disappeared.

2. The same balance of power game played by governments on an international scale.

3. These were specifically called "sex punks," and the term, "punking" meant performing anal intercourse.

4. Potrero was not yet a specialized ongoing treatment program for aggressive, poorly controlled actor-outers. Rather it was a high-turnover, temporary restraining program, sort of like a jail within the institution.

5. A favorite term in the delinquent's vocabulary, and probably *the* favorite explanation of what caused the trouble. Later, when the therapeutic community allowed free expression of humor, ward spectators at football games would sing the Youth Authority fight song, "Hey, Mess Me Over" to the tune of "Hey, Look Me Over."

6. Logic-tight compartmentalization is a mental mechanism which permits an individual to keep two diametrically opposed beliefs in his value system by never looking at the two logically side by side. A one-sentence example is, "I don't believe in capital punishment, and anyone who does should be executed."

7. The use of monitors, strong wards, as lieutenants to control the other wards by intimidation is an ancient institutional practice, and, in my opinion, a very bad one. The use of monitors was banned in the next few years, as this institution moved toward the therapeutic community approach.

8. Composed of the Assistant Superintendent, the Head Group Supervisor, and the Supervisor of Education, this body considered every case in the institution and made official recommendations to the Board regarding referral to parole. A few years later the therapeutic community ushered in the cottage case conference. This put the classification function in the hands of treatment staff, where it belonged, and permitted those high-level administrators to go do what they were supposed to do.

9. Youth authority wards were committed by the courts on indeterminant sentences, and could be paroled at any time at the discretion of the Youth Authority Board.

10. Confrontation is a vital element in the treatment of manipulative, sociopathic types.

Chapter XVI

What Is Small Group Counseling?

The following is edited from a tape-recorded dialogue between the author and a correctional worker in training. This was her first encounter with group counseling, other than having heard the term. Jane was a bright young lady who was very good at asking pertinent questions.

Bill: Good morning, Jane. We have consulted on some of your individual casework questions during the past few weeks, but now it's time to start your training in small group counseling. Here is how we are going to do it. This morning we will cover a lot of the basics. Then, I will have you sit in and observe one of my groups for a few sessions so you can see in practice the principles and techniques we have been talking about. After that, we will have another meeting to check out your experiences in my group and answer any new questions you might have thought of while observing. You probably have some questions already from having heard other counselors talking about their small groups. Where would you like to begin?

Jane: Well, maybe the first question ought to be, "Why do it at all?" What's the *purpose* of small group counseling? Does it add anything to what I can do with the kids as individuals?

Bill: Okay. Now think a minute about some of the wards you have been working with. You may have noticed that they have some things in common. One is they don't know *themselves* very well. Their self-concepts are foggy and vague. They can't define who they are except in very limited terms. They have false ideas about how other people see them, and false ideas about how other people *are* — you know, stereotypes, prejudices, and the feeling that they are all alone with their problems. Nobody else has such problems, they think. People can learn more about who they are through relating to others in a small group. They can learn first hand that others share their problems. They can learn to relate to real people, not stereotypes. They can learn how others really *do* see them. I guess a good summary of the purpose of group counseling is to help the group members, through interacting with each other, to find out who they are — to get to understand themselves and develop effective ways of relating to others.

Jane: Wow! That's a pretty big order. People get together in groups all the time, and I don't see all *those* things happening. People have bull sessions. A classroom of students is a group. There are all kinds of groups. Won't they accomplish the same things as group counseling?

Bill: Such groups can, in a haphazard way, produce a little personality growth here and there, but they aren't designed specifically for that purpose. Also, people usually think of counseling as somebody giving expert advice, like tax counseling or legal counseling. It's important to get it straight right from the beginning that *personality counseling* has absolutely nothing to do with expert advice-giving. It is a totally different process, be it group or individual, designed specifically to induce growth, self-discovery and more effective social behavior. Personality counseling itself may have a lot of different schools of thought — you know, transactional analysis, gestalt, attack therapy, and so on. In your training though, we are going to concentrate on just one approach. It is called *group-centered* counseling. It's a good place to start because it is effective in many kinds of situations, and its techniques remain useful even when the group counselor adds other systems to his bag of skills. In group-centered counseling, there is a basic assumption that the group members themselves are the ones who best know what concerns them. The group, *not* the therapy leader, decides what needs to be discussed. You see, the group leader has no power to *make* somebody grow or solve their problems. But each group member has within himself the seeds of growth—the potential for the solution of his own problems. The group leader's job is to provide the climate which will permit these seeds to grow. He does this through the way he behaves as a role model and in the way he manages the group.

Jane: What do you mean by that—the climate that will permit them to grow and solve their own problems? If they have the ability to solve their own problems, why don't they just do it? Why do they need group counseling or a special atmosphere?

Bill: Well, let's carry the seed analogy a little further. Let's say we have an acorn. Within itself the acorn has the potential ability to sprout and grow into an oak tree. But nobody can *make* it grow. We can give it advice, threaten it, or punish it for not growing, and it will just sit there, acorning away. However, if we provide the right atmosphere—rich soil, the right amounts of light, warmth and water, it will start to grow of its own accord. Then, if we attack it—freeze it, burn it, poison it, or chop on it—it will stop growing. The same is true of a person. The everyday social world is full of attacks. People criticize, "You shouldn't feel that way about it." "Shame on you for thinking such a thing." "If you believe that, you are a disgrace." What happens is that the poor guy with problems is so busy trying to defend himself against these attacks that he uses up all his growth energy. He has none left over with which to look clearly at his problems, solve them, and grow beyond them.

Jane: Well, what is different about the group counseling situation?

Bill: The group leader's job is to provide an atmosphere that encourages growth—a noncritical, non-attacking, caring relationship with the members. The message he communicates through his actions is, "I see how you feel, and you have a right to feel that way." This frees up the individual to take an objective, clear look at his own feelings and attitudes and move ahead, maybe even changing some of them as he goes.

Jane: How does the leader do this? What does he do to get the members to look at their feelings and problems?

Bill: Okay. The first thing to remember is what he doesn't do. He *never* attacks or criticizes the group members for the feelings or attitudes they express. Later, the group members will constructively criticize *each other*. This they can accept and use much better than if it came from the "authority figure." What the leader *does* is to promote *group interaction* — the expression and interchange of thoughts and feelings among the group members.

Jane: How does he do that?

Bill: His basic tools in promoting interaction are the kinds of responses he makes to the comments of the group members. Criticism, an authoritative opinion, or a long-winded speech by the leader will stop the group in its tracks. But there are certain kinds of leader responses which actively stimulate further intercommunication.

Jane: Can you describe some? What kinds of things *should* the leader say?

Bill: Okay. Let's look at a few kinds of responses that stimulate communication. We could call them techniques. First, there is reflection of a feeling or thought back to the person who expressed it. You listen carefully, then noncritically paraphrase what was said. You don't evaluate whether it was good or bad, or intelligent or dumb, or whether you agree with it or not. You just listen very carefully to make sure you understand accurately, then show that you are interested by reflecting it back in different words. Such feedback encourages the speaker to continue — to move ahead to new thoughts and feelings. As an example, you might say to me, "I'm not sure whether I want to go on and become a psychologist or quit school and take this good paying job I've been offered." To reflect this, I might say something like, "They both look good to you and you are not sure which way to go." Do you see how it works, Jane? Would you like to try one — reflecting a thought or feeling?

Jane: Okay. I think I've got the idea.

Bill: Alright. Now I'll be a member of your group, and you reflect my comment back to me. "Really, I like girls. I think about them a lot, but I get nervous when I'm around them. I'd like to get acquainted with some, but I can't get up the courage."

Jane: "Oh. You shouldn't be *afraid* of girls. They are probably as nervous as you are." Is that all right?

Bill: Sorry, Jane, but your comment was not a reflection. What it was, was a criticism, which is exactly what we should not do. You criticized me for being afraid of girls when you said, "You shouldn't feel that way." Then you threw in your own opinion about how the girls might feel, which was not a reflection of my feelings. I didn't say anything about the girls being nervous. The problem expressed was that *I* was nervous. That is what needed to be reflected. Remember, to reflect is to *paraphrase*, without agreeing, disagreeing, or throwing in your own opinion. Let's try that again. Okay?

Jane: Okay.

Bill: "I like girls, and I would like to get to know some better, but I get nervous when I think about talking to them."

Jane: "You really are interested in girls, but you are afraid to approach them."

Bill: Beautiful! Now you've got it. That was an excellent reflection of the problem I expressed. That would stimulate me to move forward with the topic. Now, let's look at another technique for stimulating communication. This one is good for bringing other group members into the exchange. We can toss an expressed idea out to the group as a whole. Following up on the same theme, the group member might say, "Yeah. I guess I am afraid. I wonder why?" The leader could stimulate more movement forward in the individual by reflecting, "You are wondering what makes you afraid of them." If, however, the leader wants to increase group interaction, he can divert the member's statement to the group, "Do any of the rest of you have any ideas on why he might be afraid to approach girls?"

Jane: Oh, I see. Sometimes maybe one person is doing all the talking, and you want to bring the others into it. So you pick out something he says, and ask the others what they think about it.

Bill: That's it exactly. Of course, sometimes the individual is really involved and needs to work on the problem some more himself, so you just continue reflecting. A good leader develops a "feeling" for when the time is right to stir up the interaction.

Jane: Okay. That's two techniques. Are there any others?

Bill: Yes. There are others. One is posing a provocative question *based on the subject under discussion*. The leader does *not* interject questions of his own choosing on unrelated subjects. As an example of this provocative question technique, suppose that a member complains because "punks" are allowed in his cottage. The leader may open up a rich exchange of opinions and feelings by asking the group, "Just what is a punk? Do we all agree on what that means?" So, there is a third technique for you – the provocative question.

Jane: It seems that all of these techniques are ways of responding to something that the group has said. So, what do you do if they don't say *anything*? What if they just sit there and look at you?

Bill: You know, that question worries a lot of people who are just starting to do group counseling. It scares them. They think, Wow! As a group leader I'm supposed to get them to talk. If they just sit there and don't say anything, I'm ruined. I'm a failure." What they don't know is that silence is itself a technique for stimulating discussion. You see, silence arouses anxiety in the group members as well as the leader, but *he* has the advantage of knowing this. The group can't stand silence for more than a few seconds. Spontaneous silences almost never last longer than half a minute, though that can seem like an hour. Often an experienced leader will deliberately remain silent and let the anxiety build until it forces out something that is bothering someone.

Jane: I would like to see these techniques in action—to see how they work in a real counseling group.

Bill: I think that is what we ought to do now, Jane. We have pretty well covered the basics of group-centered counseling. The next thing we'll do is have you sit in on a few sessions with one of my groups. I have a couple that are meeting twice a week. I'll ask the one that meets this afternoon if it's okay for you to sit in as an observer for a couple of sessions. If they agree, you can join us next week.

Jane: You have to ask your group if you can bring a visitor? I mean, you're the psychologist. It's your group, isn't it?

Bill: No, Jane. I don't see it that way. To me, "group-centered" means it's *their* group. They get to decide about and whether or not they want any outsiders to attend. Of course I've never had a group refuse to let me invite an observer for training, but it's still important to ask them. And if they said no, I'd have to find you another group. The feeling that their opinions are important, and that the group belongs to them, for *their* benefit, not mine, is an important part of the growth producing atmosphere that I'm trying to provide.

Jane: Oh. I'm beginning to see what you mean by "group-centered." You really do make the group responsible for itself. Okay. I can hardly wait to sit in.

Bill: Alright, Jane. When you are observing, what I'd like you to do is keep in mind the things we have talked about. Try to focus on my comments as leader. You might be surprised that I don't need to make very many. After a group meets a few times and the members get the hang of how it works, and what they are trying to do for each other, the group often seems to be running itself. Some of the members pick up the leader's techniques and try out the role of facilitator, or leader for themselves. This is fine. The leader just keeps quiet and let's them do it. It's good for their self-esteem. Anyway, while you are observing, pay close attention to my comments. See if you can recognize the techniques we have talked about. Also, watch for boo-boos, and watch what happens if I should goof — criticize, offer advice, or get too long-winded. You'll see the interaction come to a screeching halt.

Jane: Okay, I'll call you later today and find out about the meetings for next week.

Bill: That will be fine.

Jane sat in for three sessions as an observer in one of my groups. We then scheduled her follow-up training interview.

Bill: Well, Jane, did you get a little clearer picture of the group process — of how the leader's responses affect the interaction?

Jane: I don't know. I think I could *begin*, but I know I'd make a lot of mistakes.

Bill: Welcome to the club. I've been doing it for years, and I still make mistakes — less than I used to, though, I hope. Well, did your observation of my group raise any new questions about group counseling?

Jane: Well, it answered one. I was wondering how you arranged the group physically, but I saw that everybody sits in a circle.

Bill: Yes, and there are good reasons for doing it that way. The circle lets the leader be part of the group. It doesn't put him on a pedestal up front, like in a classroom setting. It helps to maintain the *group-centered*, as opposed to a leader-centered, atmosphere. Also it lets everybody see each other face to face. Nobody has to twist his neck turning around to look at the guy who is talking.

Jane: Of course I didn't see the first meeting. I was wondering if you have some special way of starting the group. How do you get them going in the first place?

Bill: Believe it or not, Jane, you don't really need to give any instructions to start it. I usually say something like, "Well, this is our group, and our purpose is to try to help each other. We can talk about anything you want." Then I sit back and don't say anything else until the silence anxiety forces one of the members to say something. Then I reflect it back to him, throw it out to the rest of the group, or ask a related provocative question, and we are off and running. The techniques take over from there. Of course some counselors feel uncomfortable with so little structure, so they prefer to use a catalyst technique to kick things off. There are any number of these. You can have a round robin, where you ask each member to introduce himself and tell the rest of the group a little about himself. Or, if you really need structure to allay your own anxiety, you can offer the group several topics and ask if they would like to choose one, or would they rather talk about something altogether different. You know, things like, "What causes people to get in trouble?" "What is the most terrible thing a person could do?" or, "Why do people tattoo themselves?" But, as I said, such gimmicks are unnecessary and their only value is to reassure a nervous leader who hasn't yet developed much reliance on his techniques.

Jane: Okay. Those are ways to start a group. How do you end one? Once your group is started, do you just keep on meeting week after week forever? Or how do you know when to stop?

Bill: Again, there are a number of possible approaches. You can agree upon a certain number of meetings in advance — say ten — the group to decide at the last meeting whether they have had enough or want to continue. Also, you can have either closed-ended or open ended groups. I prefer closed-ended, which doesn't permit new members to join once the group has started. This kind of group terminates by mutual agreement, or when the membership dwindles down to two or three. The open ended group replaces individual members as they leave the group. Each new member slows the progress of the more experienced ones as they have to wait for him to catch up — to get the hang of what the group process is all about. Its advantage is with a caseload such as yours, five or six kids, you can keep meeting as a group forever, replacing members as you lose them.

Jane: Those numbers raise another question. You have six wards in the group I observed. Is there anything special about that number? How many can you have in small groups?

Bill: Well, I believe that the ideal size for a small group is five to seven members. Any less than that and there isn't enough diversity of opinion to make for good interaction. Any more than seven, in my experience, the surplus members don't interact very much. With, say ten wards, what you get is six or seven actively participating, and the rest just kind of sitting there vegetating.

Jane: Your meetings were fifty minutes long. Is that standard?

Bill: That's a good length for most Youth Authority wards, but it kind of depends on the maturity level and attention spans of the members. Some can't handle more than half an hour. Others can interact productively for over an hour. One thing I would advise is, once you have agreed on the length of the meetings, don't go into overtime. Stop each meeting right on time, no matter how involved and exciting the discussion is. There are a couple of reasons for this. One is that the members will carry the excitement and anxiety out of the meeting with them, and the therapeutic process will continue to operate between then and the next meeting. If you keep the meeting going until a resolution is reached, this continuation of the therapeutic process will not occur. In group counseling, we are not seeking resolutions and conclusions. Another reason to end the meetings promptly is that, if you don't, group members tend to stall and avoid getting down to business until just a few minutes remain. The meetings get longer and longer. Ending promptly encourages them to start "working" earlier at the next session.

Jane: How often should a group meet?

Bill: At least once a week. I prefer twice, or even three times with some groups. Less than once a week will not let the continuity develop that produces growth.

Jane: One last question, Bill. Do you think I am ready to start doing group with my caseload? Is it safe without more training?

Bill: Well, Jane, as you know, I run several counseling groups for staff who are doing group counseling with wards. We focus on their group counseling experiences and problems. I would like you to get into one of these staff groups. That way we can continue with your training, and work through any problem you may run into with your group of wards. But yes, Jane. You *can* safely use the techniques we have discussed here. Go ahead. Get your feet wet!

Chapter XVII

A Group-Centered Experience

Each of the wards who formed this group came to me at his own request for individual counseling. As I perceived that an intensive small group interaction experience would be the treatment of choice for each of them, I explained small group counseling, asked if they would be interested, and said I would keep their names on file until we had enough to form a group. One criterion for their selection was diversity of personality types and social status in the institution.

J.D. Boothe was a bright, very verbal, sixteen-year-old who had achieved the rank of "Punk" in the social hierarchy. He's bitter because, ". . . so many guys act like they are hot shit, even though they are a lot dumber than me." J.D. rarely spoke a sentence that was not punctuated by one or more obscenities.

Jim Caven, fifteen, was in a Straight firm. He enjoyed his anti-authority attitude, and loved to expound on it. He was concerned about his status in a rejecting family, but avoided the subject in the presence of his peers, opting for the role of super-cool straight stud.

Lenny Coyle, glib, smooth-talking Blood firm member was seventeen. He maintained a surface devil-may-care attitude, and was adept at controlling conversations by playing word games and leading people astray, so as to avoid facing real issues. My first impression was that he was struggling with some kind of sexual identity conflict.

Del Swanson, seventeen, was quiet, withdrawn, and a loner. He had been diagnosed by Clinic staff as a schizoid personality. His initial complaint to me was that he had no friends. Socially, he was considered by his peers to fall somewhere between Punk and Semistraight, but they weren't quite sure where he fit because he was kind of big and never said anything to anybody, so they just left him alone.

Pat Muldoon, homely, rawboned, muscular, and the biggest youngster in the group at six feet, 180 pounds was, if anything, quieter than Swanson. His demeanor, however, was vastly different. While Swanson appeared bland and emotionless, Muldoon seethed with unspoken anger. For several sessions at the beginning, Pat just sat listening and glaring, his face actually turning purple, without uttering a word.[1] He complained that he didn't like anybody. He was a sixteen-year-old Semi-straight loner. His peers didn't dare classify Pat as a Punk because he was just too big, strong, ugly and mean-looking.

SESSION #1 NOTES

The primary theme was angry criticism of authority in general, and institutional staff and procedures in particular.[2] Coyle, Caven and Boothe did all the talking. I simply reflected the expressed feelings back to the speaker or tossed them back to the rest of the group. Interaction was lively among the three. Muldoon just sat glowering, and Swanson just sat. Neither said a word.

Toward the end of the session, Boothe, loud and profane, cursed people who said things that reflect on his mother. He kept referring to them as "those bastards" and "those motherfuckers." Finally, Jim Caven had enough and pointed out that J.D. was calling these people the very names that he objected to being called himself. "You don't know *their* mothers any more than they know yours." Boothe didn't curse for a while, and refrained entirely from using "mother" terms for the rest of the hour.

SESSION #2 NOTES

Lenny Coyle took control of the group immediately by posing his own provocative question, "What can be done about two guys who love each other so much that one of them doesn't want to leave the institution without the other?" The rest of the group took the bait and spent the entire session playing a variation of twenty questions, trying to coax Coyle into revealing the identities of his mystery lovers. Eventually I tried to shift the focus by asking Coyle what there was about this situation that made it so interesting to him. He evaded the question and countered with one of his own, "Can they be helped if they don't want help?" The session was not very productive, except toward the end Caven and Boothe started to show a little annoyance, as if they were catching on to the game Coyle was running on them. Our two silent members remained silent.

SESSION #3 NOTES

Del Swanson was absent. He asked to be excused before the meeting started ". . . to catch up on some school work."

Lenny began another mystery, this time about some vague person in a vague place, whom he, very soon, will "have to go see." The group began to "bite," and Lenny became evasive, grinning and declining to answer their questions. I confronted[3] him, "Is this a problem that you feel we might help you with, or do you just enjoy taking the group on a wild-goose chase? Our purpose here really is not to play guessing games or to try to solve mysteries." J.D. Boothe echoed my sentiment that we have had enough of word games. Coyle dropped the subject.

Jim Caven began to complain about inconsistencies and injustices perpetrated on wards by institutional staff. He mentioned subjective grading based on personal feelings. Coyle and Boothe chimed in and registered a number of other complaints. The emotional tone was more grumbly than vehement, until suddenly, with a lion-like roar, Pat Muldoon unleashed his first words since joining the group, "The only thing you have to do to get out of here is kiss all the supervisors' asses!" The startled group applauded. Pat grinned, leaned back and resumed his silence.

Near closing time, Jim Caven complained that supervisors are prejudiced against "Straight firm" members. "Like hell they are!" objected J.D. Boothe angrily. "Those guys can get away with anything because the supervisors don't want to make them salty. It's the guys out in the middle[4] that can't do anything." Jim looked startled at Boothe's audacity, as he was unaccustomed to being addressed in this fashion by a Punk. However, he did not reply, and switched to a different complaint.

SESSION #4 NOTES

Del Swanson returned to the group, but said nothing for the entire session. He has yet to make a comment in the group.

Jim Caven introduced the topic of premarital sex by stating that, since most people do it, the law ought to allow it. This theme was immediately dismissed by Lennie Coyle, who asked an irrelevant question about his status regarding parole. I told him that he can get that information from his Classification Counselor, and asked the group if they would like to continue with Jim's topic. The three talkers addressed it briefly, basically agreeing with Jim's original statement.

J.D. Boothe said that he wanted to hear the others' ideas about "Punks." This opened up a rich discussion of what Punks are, who says so, how they are selected for that status, and whether there really is such a class of people, or if they are just made up by some other people trying to make themselves feel important. The exchange of views among "Straight-stud" Caven, "Blood" Coyle and "Punk" Boothe was active and heated. All three, however, displayed courtesy and tolerance toward each other's positions. I summarized by citing the principle that words are merely symbols and have no absolute meanings. "Symbols only represent things. They are *not themselves* the things they represent. Since we can use a word to represent anything we want it to, in communicating it is often wise to define what we mean when we use a word, rather than falsely assume that it means the same thing to everybody. 'Punk' is a good example."

SESSION #5 NOTES

Del Swanson asked for, and received permission to be excused to do some school work. He seems to be gaining something of value from the mere act of deciding for himself whether or not to attend. (A little exercise in independence?)

Lennie Coyle attempted to seize control of the meeting by vaguely referring to his personal problems in areas about which the group had no information. I suggested that if he wanted to make a group topic of whatever it was he was referring to, he should provide some details so the other members would know what he was talking about. He fell silent.

Jim Caven complained about the unfairness of statutory rape laws, opining that age fourteen would be more sensible than eighteen as a legal age of consent. Coyle and Boothe joined him in a heated discussion of inconsistencies in the laws governing sex. I attempted to arouse some constructive thinking by asking, "Do you think the statutory rape law has any purpose or value at all?" Jim, Lennie and J.D., however, were far too busy expressing their sexual frustrations to be sidetracked. Pat Muldoon listened in silence.

SESSION #6 NOTES

Del Swanson returned.

Also present was Mr. X., Senior Group Supervisor of one of the living units. Mr. X. is observing as part of his group counseling training. He plans to have his staff trained also, and provide small group opportunities for all the wards in his cottage.

The group was mute for almost half a minute, probably due to Mr. X.'s presence, although they had been prepared for it. Finally, as I let the silence continue, it became too much for Coyle to bear. He suggested that we continue with Caven's topic of premarital sex and the statutory rape law. The group, except for Swanson and Muldoon who remained quiet as usual, took up the suggestion and began propounding free sex. Their language was far more obscene than usual, again probably due to Mr. X.'s presence. They seemed to be trying to get across the message that even though he was a Senior Supervisor, and prohibited such language on his living unit, he had no power to tell them how to talk in *their* group. Mr. X. ignored the purple language.

Jim Caven again pointed out that to a teenage boy, fifteen, sixteen, seventeen and eighteen-year-old girls are very similar and that the legal age of consent, arbitrarily set at eighteen, is ridiculous.

Fifteen, he said, would make a lot more sense. Coyle and Boothe enthusiastically voiced their agreement. Muldoon, and even Swanson, nodded in approval. This time, however, when I asked if there might be any purpose or value in the statutory rape law, J.D. Boothe said, "Sure. It protects little children from nasty adults." The others agreed, and decided that the law shouldn't be abolished entirely—just modified to make sense.

J.D. asked what the others thought caused delinquency. Lennie attacked neglectful parents as the culprits, without naming any particulars. Jim used himself as evidence contradictory to Lennie's view. He pointed out that his parents had planned with him to get a car. In fact, they actually got him one on the day after, unknown to them, he had stolen one for a "joy ride." On the third day the police picked him up. Boothe opined that schools contributed a lot to producing delinquency. Both Caven and Coyle agreed, admitting that they had a need for much stronger external controls than the public schools had provided. I asked, "If nobody provides controls from the outside, then what?" Boothe said, "Maybe you have to learn to control yourself." Pat Muldoon (yes, Silent Muldoon) said, "Or the Youth Authority will do it for you."

SESSION #7 NOTES

Senior Supervisor, Mr. X., was again present.

Lennie and J.D. did most of the talking today. It was difficult to identify a theme due to Coyle's rambling ideation which somehow manages to reach the topic of homosexuality, no matter what the starting point. Intermingled in the confused flow of Coyle's speech were points related to stealing, which Boothe kept trying to discuss. He was propounding a Robin Hood type philosophy that it is all right to steal from fat cats and give the loot to folks who need it more. Every time the group showed interest in this theme, Coyle short circuited it.

One other theme which tried to emerge, the effects of false rumors and gossip on wards, was also nipped in the bud by Lennie Coyle's persistent marching to a different drummer. At one point I asked him how he managed to get so quickly from the topic of stealing to "sucking dicks." He tried to relate the two logically, but became confused.

SESSION #8 NOTES

Lennie Coyle brought up, strangely, one of the topics that he cut off at the last meeting, rumors and gossip. The group kicked it around for a while, agreeing that the effects on the victim can be devastating, be he ward or staff. Several examples were cited.

J.D. Boothe complained about the censoring of wards' mail and other restrictive institutional practices. The group discussed these issues at some length, and, surprisingly ended up siding with administration.[5] They brought out a number of reasons why such regulations were necessary. They concluded that the irresponsible actions of a few individuals make these rigid practices necessary for the whole ward population.

Prompted by a direct question from Mr. X., Del Swanson spoke for the first time as a member of the group. To everyone's surprise, he spoke eloquently, summarizing the conclusions reached by the others regarding the necessity for institutional regulations.

Perhaps inspired by Swanson, even Pat Muldoon made several comments.

The closing minutes were devoted to a discussion of the severe punishments and terrible conditions imposed upon prisoners in various jails and juvenile halls. Expressing anger toward certain peers who make life miserable for him, Del Swanson declared that these highly punitive facilities are just perfect for "certain mess-ups," and they ought to be sent there.

SESSION #9 NOTES

This was Mr. X.'s last meeting as an observer. He is now ready to start his own group.

Del Swanson was absent, ill in the infirmary.

Lennie Coyle began with a description of sexual activities on his cottage, making it sound like a homosexual Peyton Place. The others, except for Muldoon, continued on this theme. Coyle's view was that sexual expression of some kind is an absolute necessity, and that people will take whatever is available to them. He said that he thinks sex punks are homosexuals, but the straight studs who punk them are not. J.D. Boothe differed. He felt that the degree of sexual need depended upon the individual. Further, he stated that the two males are both "mentally off," the one who gives it and the one who gets it from a boy. He closed the discussion with the opinion that there ought to be at least two staff on duty at all times to prevent such sexual activities from happening.

Today's meeting involved much less obscene language than has been the case since Mr. X. began observing.

SESSION #10 NOTES

Jim Caven expressed anger toward authority, ranging from his school teacher who sent him to Potrero this week to the entire government of the State of California. I reflected remarks until he got a lot of the negative feelings out of his system, then tossed the theme out to the group as a whole. The entire group, *including Swanson and Muldoon*, interacted well in the discussion that followed. I summarized and added that there seemed to be two aspects to the problem. One is that society really does impose some unnecessary and unfair sanctions. The other was the difference between individuals in their ability to adjust to this. Some are able to get along all right, rolling with the punches when necessary, but maintaining a pretty good working relationship with the rest of society. Others can't seem to do this, and constantly alienate themselves and blame society for their troubles. I asked, "Why can many people live in, and be happy as part of society, and others can't seem to accomplish this?" Jim Caven noted defensively that the institution is a far cry from real society.

The group picked up this theme, and again had a good interaction session with all members participating. They concluded that the criteria by which wards are deemed ready for release are largely unrelated to their real potential for success on parole. "Hell," said Muldoon, "at home I'm not going to get my parole revoked for talking on silence or marching out of step."

SESSION #11 NOTES

Del Swanson asked why a person would try to kill himself. I asked why he asked. He designated J.D. Boothe as his referent. Boothe cut his wrist in a non-dangerous area a few days ago. The group discussed the incident, concluding that he had not really meant to kill himself, but was trying to attract attention or sympathy. Boothe protested. Caven asked him why he had cut where the veins weren't. Boothe said that he thought there might be some veins up higher (about mid-forearm) where he cut (scratched, actually). The group was not convinced of the sincerity of Boothe's suicidal intent. He realized this and didn't push the issue any further.

With full interaction, the group went on to discuss the stupidity of suicide, pointing out that problems which might make one contemplate it can usually be resolved by talking them out with someone. Numerous other constructive approaches to problem solving exist, and ought to be exhausted before suicide is considered, they said.

The entire group then denounced impulsive behavior of any kind, and stressed the necessity to consider consequences as a mature approach to choice of action. All members admitted having been too impulsive in the past, and claimed to be learning to think and evaluate possible consequences before acting.

They moved from suicide to capital punishment, discussing it pro and con. They concluded that it is ineffective at deterring crimes of passion, illogical, and probably in opposition to the laws of God.

Final theme for the day was the group's perception that state institutions are needed for the care and treatment of the unfortunate inhabitants of skid rows. Each member expressed his sympathy for these people, blind beggars and others who are down and out. Each declared that he always gives them his last dime. Muldoon said, "There are probably a lot of boys in here who stole things from rich people to give the poor ones." "Yeah," said J.D., "like Robin Hood." I asked how many of the boys in here that they know personally, actually gave the things they stole to the poor. Coyle said, "None." The group laughed and agreed. They had reached the conclusion that the Robin Hood myth is a myth.

SESSION #12 NOTES

Jim Caven delivered a tirade against the Senior Supervisor on his living unit, citing several instances of bullying, dictatorial, unfair and discriminatory behavior. Then he described with pride some of his own manipulative behavior, getting away with all kinds of skull-duggery, only to be blamed for something he didn't do, which he considered grossly unfair. He was very bitter about the extreme regimentation and "meaningless discipline" imposed by his Senior Supervisor. He astutely observed that because of this, the angry wards took it out on weaker staff when the "strong" Senior was away.

The group returned to the theme of the artificiality of the institutional environment, and how it renders the criteria for parole readiness meaningless. All members took turns asking questions such as, "When will we get graded down at home for talking on silence?" "Will mother give us a grade down for smoking in the latrine?" "Will there be a grade down on the outs for not marching right?" "Will we get graded down for passing food at the dinner table at home?" "Will we get graded down for not going to the latrine when someone tells us to even though we already went and don't have to?" I summarized in a reflection, "You feel that the things you are graded on here to determine your readiness for release are not related to real life on the outs." Jim Caven said, "Yeah. They say that learning to obey these little rules will make you obey the big rules on the outs. That's a bunch of shit! These things don't have anything to do with that. You don't mind so much if rules have some real purpose. But these don't have any."

SESSION #13 NOTES

Dr. Y., staff physician is observing, not because he intends to do group counseling, but just because he wants to learn something of what it is about.

The major portion of the meeting was a medical question and answer program, stimulated by Dr. Y.'s presence.

A little interaction developed toward the end of the hour. J.D. Boothe told several tales about how he had saved lives in medical emergencies, and refused anesthetics when he required surgery.

Lennie Coyle suggested that Boothe should leave the practice of medicine to the professionals who are trained and licensed to do it. J.D. didn't respond, and nobody else jumped in, so I said, "J.D., it seems that you enjoy placing yourself in a hero's role, doing something dramatic or brave." He was embarrassed, but accepted the interpretation with no more than a blush and a, "Well, God damn!"

SESSION #14 NOTES

Dr. Y. was present again. He began the session by asking Coyle about his earache. Lennie reported it improved.

I asked the group, "Where shall we begin today?" trying to forestall another medical question and answer period. Several individuals made self-centered comments, all lacking general interest. Each comment was ignored by the others. Eventually Jim Caven drew the group's attention by describing a dream that he was an atomic bomb that exploded when a doctor was about to operate on him. I asked the group what feelings this dream seemed to express. Muldoon said, "Mentally disturbed." Nobody could offer anything more specific, so I suggested that maybe Jim felt like "blowing up"—that perhaps the dream reflected anger. Jim quickly denied this, stating that he never gets angry. He said that he laughs all the time, even when he is hurting somebody. He gave examples of fights during which he laughed and felt no anger while he was beating somebody up. I interpreted, "Since you felt no anger toward the ones you were hurting, maybe you were in fact mad at somebody else and taking it out on the wrong targets." J.D. Boothe interpreted, "He's a sadistic bastard!" Jim ignored Boothe, and admitted that he does get angry at staff, but knows better than to express directly his feelings to them, so he just smiles and goes along with them. I said, "You hurt people you are not mad at, and are nice and polite to the ones who do make you mad." Jim said, "Yeah. That's not right, is it?" J.D. said, "Hell no."

Several other dreams were reported, but before any discussion of any one of them could take place, another member would jump in with another dream.

Finally the topic switched to eating and sleeping habits. Pat Muldoon reported that he thrived on twelve or thirteen hours of sleep and one meal per day. Jim Caven said that he didn't require more than six or seven hours sleep, but ate that many meals per day, and was still always hungry. The group recognized that such individual differences make for real problems and frustrations in a regimented program. Caven always had to be lying in bed hungry when he wanted to be eating while Muldoon had to be up all day eating when he wasn't hungry and wanted to be sleeping.

Little Boothe, with his flair for the dramatic, claimed that at home he always ate three or four huge steaks for breakfast, along with a few cans of beer. Del Swanson said, "You probably never saw a can of beer in your life." Muldoon added, "He just likes to play hero." Boothe was squelched. He recognized that his immature status seeking play was not successful, but took it good-naturedly.

SESSION #15 NOTES

Caven, Muldoon and Boothe took turns relating the details of their apprehension by the police. Boothe's account sounded kind of feeble and childish by comparison to the daring exploits of the other two.

The theme shifted to the wild and reckless driving of the group members' parents. Each told exaggerated humorous anecdotes. Boothe told the group how he used to fantasize, while riding with his parents, that he was a tail gunner shooting down hundreds of enemy planes.

J.D. told the group about the book he is writing and tried to heighten their interest in it by stressing that it contains sex. This *was* interesting, at least to Lennie Coyle.

After the meeting, Boothe asked if I could see him individually as well as in the group. I told him that my schedule is completely filled, but I will put him on the waiting list.

SESSION #16 NOTES

For various reasons, only Muldoon and Boothe were present. I asked them if they would like to skip it today, or have me tell them some things about how people's minds work. They chose the latter.

I talked to them about mental defense mechanisms, emphasizing the ones upon which Boothe depends too much, though not identifying them as such. He recognized, nonetheless, that they were his. He squirmed, took exception, rationalized, and denied. Each time he used one of these mechanisms, I pointed it out as a good example of what I was explaining. One mechanism which seemed to have an especially meaningful impact on Boothe was "substitution," as when people substitute obscene language for real sexuality.

While Muldoon listened quietly with no comment, Boothe surprised me at the end of the session by volunteering, "This was cool. We ought to do it again. It was really interesting."

SESSION #17 NOTES

This was Dr. Y.'s last day as an observer.

Destructive behavior was the major theme. Each member described wild Halloween adventures and other destructive "kicks" they had enjoyed in the past. Boothe accused Caven of being "pretty low," wanting to beat up his girlfriend, since girls should be respected and protected. Caven boasted about his disregard for all convention and lack of feeling for people he hurts. He described himself as cold-blooded. I said, "It kind of protects you and lets you do anything you want to people if you bury your feelings and pretend you don't have any." He looked startled and didn't reply.

J.D. Boothe interrupted Del Swanson several times when Del was trying to tell about his prowess as a baseball pitcher. Finally Del demanded, "Will you keep quiet a minute? I'm trying to say something."[6] Boothe mumbled briefly, then kept quiet.

When Swanson finished describing his pitching ability, Boothe asked me, "From all the times you have seen me, what do you think is wrong with me?" I said, "Since this is a group meeting, maybe the group ought to take up your question." He started to disapprove of this idea but it was too late, as the group eagerly grabbed at the opportunity to tell J.D. what was wrong with him. Swanson said, "I know." Caven said, "Go ahead, Professor. Tell him what his problems are." Swanson accused Boothe of having no interest in, or respect for, anybody but himself. He cited J.D.'s repeated interruptions and blatant lack of courtesy as examples. Boothe sputtered. I reflected Swanson's statement back to him, "You feel that J.D. thinks only of himself, and doesn't care anything about others." Caven added, "Yeah, and he's always giving us that Robin Hood shit—steal from the rich and give to the poor. Crap! He don't care about the poor, or anybody else."

Self-destructive play, like "chicken" and Russian Roulette became the topic. The group recited a number of such games they have played, each trying to be more blood curdling than the others. I raised the question, "Why do you suppose some people enjoy playing those games?" The group couldn't come up with any answers more profound than, "For kicks." I said, "It seems to me that people who have to go about proving their courage in this way must really have some strong doubts about their strength and bravery. A truly self-confident man would laugh at such antics as childish, stupidly dangerous, and a waste of time, since he already *knows* he is a man." The group accepted my comment without defensiveness.

Caven condemned one of his supervisors for having given him a grade down for "bad attitude." Coyle said, "Yeah. But the problem is that your attitude really is bad."

After the meeting Boothe lingered to tell me that he had learned something from Del Swanson's analysis of his self-centeredness. He assured me, however, using extremely vile language as a couple of female staff members passed by, that he really does respect other people's feelings. I asked, "Like those ladies' feelings about your language?" He looked at them retreating down the hall and actually blushed. He had been oblivious to the situation. He said that he was beginning to learn some things about himself.

SESSION #18 NOTES

Del Swanson and Lennie Coyle have been paroled. Jim Caven asked to be excused to go swimming.

Muldoon and Boothe chatted about impersonal things such as the destructive power of nuclear weapons, and speculated as to whether an ice cube with mile long sides could be cut out of the polar ice cap with an acetylene torch.

I suggested that, with our group down to three, maybe we should consider terminating. I said that we can talk about it next time.

SESSION #19 NOTES

Boothe was away on a trip to the beach. I told Muldoon and Caven that we don't have enough members left for group meetings and I think that it is time for us to disband. I already have Boothe in individual therapy. I offered to continue to meet with Caven and Muldoon individually if they wanted to do it. Muldoon accepted. Caven declined, saying that he didn't need it.

CONCLUSION

Swanson, Muldoon and Boothe all showed outstanding social and emotional growth as members of this small group. While such change was not obvious in Coyle and Caven, the group gave them a place to verbalize their angry and antisocial feelings, rather than acting them out in other areas of their programs and getting in more trouble.

Moral: Group-centered counseling has a dual purpose. It is therapeutic; and it is an excellent management tool for impulsive and hostile types.

NOTES

1. Remarkably, some months later, as a result of this group experience and a transfer into Escalon, Pat became a warm, good natured young man with many friends. Subsequently, he made an outstanding post-institutional adjustment.

2. This is often the early theme of small groups. One reason is that institutional staff *do* a lot of things that generate anger. Another is that the members want to test the leader to see if he will come to the defense of the institution and censure them for their attitudes. Is it really *their* group, or a pro-authority sham?

3. Confrontation is not a technique which fits comfortably into the group-centered philosophy; but occasionally it is necessary to wrest control of the group from a self-centered manipulator and return it to the other members.

4. Firm members commandeered all the seating areas around the dayroom perimeter, considered most desirable. Punks had to sit out in the middle.

5. Apparently some maturation has taken place in the group. There is no way this bunch of renegades could have taken a pro-authority position on anything when we started.

6. This was a remarkable display of ego strength for a young man who was unable to utter a word in the group until the eighth meeting.

Chapter XVIII

Behind The Back:
A Special Kind
of Small Group Therapy
Designed Specifically to Correct
Discrepancies in the Self-Concept

Often the difficulties encountered by delinquent youth are rooted in some kind of discrepancy between the individuals' self-concept and reality. Several variables are involved. One is how he sees himself. Another is how he would like to see himself (ideal self-image). Another is how he thinks other people see him. Finally, is how others really do see him.

A happy, socially well-adjusted person is one whose image of himself closely approximates what he would like to be, and whose beliefs regarding how others view him are quite close to how they really do perceive him. If he sees himself as a far cry from what he would like to be, he will feel frustrated and inferior. If others' views of him are greatly different from what he thinks they are, his behavior toward them will be inappropriate and self-defeating. Put these together and they make a pretty good definition of a juvenile delinquent, i.e., a young person often characterized by feelings of frustration and inferiority, and by inappropriate antisocial behavior toward others.

A review of the preceding chapter reveals a number of instances in which group-centered counseling produced corrections of these kinds of discrepancies (e.g., when the group let J.D. Boothe know he wasn't fooling them with his heroic lies). On the one hand, such corrections *are* made in group-centered counseling, but they are scattered, and are incidental to the flow of the group process. The "Behind the Back" method featured in this chapter, on the other hand, is aimed specifically at correcting self-concept discrepancies. It gets right to the point.

Members for such a group are selected because they show inferiority feelings or play phony, inappropriate roles in relating to others, or both. I'll introduce the cast of this play in a minute, but first I'll describe the method.

No. First, I'll describe *why* the method. When folks are face to face discussing each other they lie a lot. When they talk about the same person to their neighbor across the fence (gossip), they tell the truth.

Why? When we are eyeball-to-eyeball, we are afraid to speak the truth. (This dude might be dangerous, if confronted.) When we hear somebody say something *about* us, instead of *to* us, we believe it, because the image wall is down, and we accept it as how people *really* see us when they are not trying to be polite.

Thus, in behind-the-back counseling, the situation is structured so that the group focuses on one individual at a time while he is sitting behind them, with his back to their backs, so they cannot see each other. The leader sits in front of the semicircle so that he sees the faces of the discussants and the back of the head of the discussee.

The discussee, technically, is called the "subject" of the meeting, but in every such group I have conducted, after a few sessions, the members have started (good naturedly) referring to the subject as the victim, as in, "Well, who is going to be the victim at our next meeting?"

At the end of each meeting one of the members volunteers to be the subject of the next session. His intensive self-image therapy begins right then. He is greatly concerned about how the others will treat him when he is on the hot seat. He spends a great deal of his time after volunteering wondering if he should have, who he is, who he would like to be, how he should present himself to the group, and what they will think of him. By the time his meeting actually materializes, he has already come to grips with the fact that his self-concept is uncertain and that he has grave doubts about how he impresses others. This is the first step toward making some corrections and developing a self-concept that is more compatible with external reality. I prefer to have behind-the-back groups meet no more frequently than once per week in order to give this introspection process time to work.

Some subjects, those with severely battered self-esteem, approach their meetings with great fear that they will be crushed by rejection. Others, whose ego balloons are overinflated, come in expecting to con the group with their super-cool acts and receive the adulation they think they deserve. Members of a behind-the-back group invariably show amazing sensitivity, giving tremendous support to the poor guy that needs it, and sticking pins in the bloated ego balloons that need puncturing.

The behind-the-back meeting itself is divided into four parts, roughly equal, time-wise. In a one-hour meeting the following segments are allotted about fifteen minutes each:

1. The volunteer subject, sitting in the semicircle facing the others, talks about himself. He can talk about his hopes, fears, experiences, problems, love life, or whatever he chooses, as long as it is focused on himself. He may not wander into current events, politics, sports, or other topics that are unrelated to him as a person. During this period the leader or the other members may reflect the subject's feelings or ask him questions for clarification purposes. They may *not* state opinions, evaluate aloud, or make interpretations of the subject's remarks. It is the leader's job to enforce these ground rules.

2. The second portion is the behind-the-back segment. The leader instructs the subject to move his chair behind the semicircle and sit with his back to the others. The subject is told, "You are going away so the group will be able to talk about you with complete honesty. They want to discuss what kind of a guy you really are, and they couldn't be completely open and honest about that if you were sitting here looking at them."

When the subject has moved to behind-the-back, the leader addresses the others, "Okay, _____ has gone away. I want you to think of him as being in another room, or returned to his cottage. He is not here. He cannot hear you. You remember from when we talked about it individually, the only way this group can help anybody is by being completely frank and honest. We are going to talk about _____ while he is not here. What we are after is truth. What kind of a guy is _____, really? What was he telling you about himself? What do you think of him?" At this point the group discusses _____, just as if he really were not there. The leader reflects feelings and in other ways stimulates group interaction in the discussion. He also jots down on a piece of paper the salient points hit upon by the group.

This method, by breaking the eye contact, does a couple of amazing things. It lets the group be completely candid in their comments about the subject; and it lets the subject accept these comments from people he can't see without having to jump up and pop somebody on the nose (which I have seen happen in group-centered sessions).

3. In the third portion the leader calls the subject back into the semicircle and tells him, "While you were away the group had a little talk about you. I thought you might be interested in what they had to say, so sit down and I'll tell you." Then the leader, referring to his notes, summarizes the points made by the group. Thus, the subject receives a double dose of the same insights, once behind-the-back from his peers, and once again from an authority figure, face-to-face. (Also, the subject can't very well become defensive with the authority figure, since he is merely reporting what the group said.)

After the leader's summary, he says to the subject, "Well, that's what the group had to say about you. How does it strike you? Is there anything you would like to say in response?" The rest of this segment then belongs to the subject. He is free to agree or disagree with points made by the group, laugh, cry, become defensive, or respond in any other way he chooses (except with physical violence).

4. Segment four is group-centered, with the subject interacting with the rest of the group. Here they are free to ask questions, clarify their statements, argue about them, or whatever.

At the end of the meeting, the leader asks for a volunteer to be subject of the next meeting. At the beginning of the next meeting, the preceding subject is usually asked for a brief retrospective comment on his experience.

A BEHIND-THE-BACK-EXPERIENCE

Each member of this group was selected from a different living unit. Let's meet them as individuals.

Bud Bush is an unstable fifteen-year-old whose history includes many encounters with the law for malicious mischief, assault, burglary, lack of parental control, and various sexual misadventures. He has performed oral copulation with males a number of times, but has also enjoyed heterosexual experiences. He seems motivated to reduce the effeminate components of his personality, but is deterred by his relationship with his mother, and desertion by his alcoholic father when Bud's mother fell ill three years ago. The mother, still physically frail, is highly competitive, demanding, especially toward Bud, and seems confused about her own psychosexual role. Bud admits to having sexual fantasies about her.

Glen Grant is sixteen, five feet three inches tall, and has no record of delinquency prior to his commitment offense, which was theft of a revolver. He told the court that he stole the gun with the intention of shooting a twenty-three-year-old divorcee who dumped him after a brief sexual affair. Glen confided to me that this is not the true story. In fact, he stole the gun to protect himself from his own stepfather, who was also lusting after the divorcee, and threatened to kill Glen after he discovered that he had had sex with her. Glen said that he lied to the court because his stepfather was on parole from prison and might have been sent back had Glen told the truth.

Mickey Switt is a relatively normal fifteen-year-old. He is hostile toward authority, and expresses it in passive ways such as sneaky malicious mischief and burglary of unoccupied residences. When one victim returned home unexpectedly, however, Mickey threatened him with a revolver, bound him, and escaped. He is passive-aggressively dragging his anchor in the institutional program, making no progress toward earning his parole.

Floyd Walters, seventeen, exudes so much loneliness that it hurts those around him. His hair and skin are so white that he would be an albino if his eyes were pink rather than pale blue. Floyd came to see me to express despair about his severe acne. He says that he will not go home until his face gets well because his father attacks him about it. His father tells Floyd that it is his own fault, and accuses him of not washing his face. Floyd scrubs it several times a day. He avoids looking in mirrors because he can't stand to see himself. He was committed to the Youth Authority for petty theft. His only prior offense was running away from home.

Warren Krist is a fifteen-year-old from a wealthy family, committed for burglary. His childhood history of poor health contributed to a pattern of maternal overprotection. Resenting this role, Warren has combined genius-level intelligence and an interest in physical science in his protest. His "practical jokes," some of which contributed to his commitment to the Youth Authority, included making explosives in his home chemistry lab and setting them off around the neighborhood; constructing a flamethrower and burning down the hedges at a public school with it; and wiring the toilet in his home so he could, by remote control, shock his mother's party guests. He told me, grinning, that the toilet "experiment" was an especially good one. Three years ago he underwent three months of private psychotherapy, at which time it was terminated, his therapist noting that no progress was being made.

SESSION #1 NOTES

I had the members introduce themselves. Then I explained again in detail how the behind-the-back method works, although I had gone over it earlier with each of them in individual interviews.

The remainder of the hour was thrown open to group-centered discussion. Typically, they used it to test the situation and me by expressing contempt for the institution and staff, and trying out some profanity. Group morale was high at the end of the session.

Glen Grant volunteered to be the subject of our next meeting.

SESSION #2 NOTES

Glen Grant, today's subject, told the group that his problem seemed to be "always losing." He described his affair with the twenty-three-year-old divorcee, his stepfather's reaction, and the other circumstances leading to his incarceration, always with an air of boastfulness.

He modestly hinted at his brilliance, stating that he used to be an expert on nuclear physics, and then lost this knowledge as a result of the family trauma. This was another illustration, he said, of "always losing." (His school records show no background in math or basic science.)

In the behind-the-back phase, the group attacked Glen's character defense point-blank, but in a matter-of-fact, nonhostile way. He heard himself described as someone who ". . . pretends he knows more than he really does." The group said that he "always loses" because he is always trying to prove that he can do things that he really cannot. As an example, the group felt that his Youth Authority commitment stemmed from his trying to prove that he was as big a man as his stepfather. They added that Glen's constant need to prove how great he is probably comes from feelings about his small physical size.

The group said that Glen's stepfather had taunted him, casting aspersions upon his ability to have an affair with a woman, and Glen reacted to the challenge wildly and impulsively.

Supportively then, the group noted that Glen is quite intelligent and has the ability to become, as he grows up, a *real* "big wheel" and contribute something to the world. To do this, however, he must channel his talents into more stable and constructive activities and quit trying to fool people about how much he knows, and stop striking out blindly on escapades such as he described, in attempting to prove himself a man. They emphasized that consistent hard work, not wishful fantasy, is what underlies *real* accomplishment.

I ended the behind-the-back phase, and recalled Glen to the group. Referring to my notes, I told him again face-to-face, how the group had evaluated him and his problems. Then I advised him that it was his turn to respond to what they had said about him in any way that he chose.

Glen first stated that the group had "hit the nail on the head," then spent the rest of his rebuttal period making not very convincing explanations, attempting to negate the group's analysis.

In the final open discussion phase Glen reverted to his boastful pretending. He tried to impress the group by alluding to his alleged expertise regarding nuclear physics. Bush responded, demonstrating that he is at least as knowledgeable as Glen in this area. Finally,

Warren Krist had heard enough of this amateurish prattle, and ended the debate by describing in some detail how to build a cyclatron.[1]

Warren Krist volunteered to be next week's subject.

SESSION #3 NOTES

When asked to reflect on his experience as last week's subject, Glen Grant reported that he has thought a lot about what the group said, and has concluded that they were pretty accurate.

Today's subject, Warren Krist, revealed to the group that his mother had always overprotected him because of his poor health as a child. He also told us that he has a younger brother whose hobby is electronic musical instruments, building and playing them. His brother, Warren said, has always been "babied too much."

The remainder of his presentation Warren devoted to a bland, almost emotionless account of a number of his "practical jokes," including some that I hadn't heard or read about in his files. For instance, he manufactured hydrogen in his lab, inflated six feet-in-diameter balloons with it, and released them at night with long, burning fuses attached. They soared high over the city and exploded in great flashes of light, prompting a flood of calls to official agencies with questions and reported sightings of everything from flying saucers to alien airplanes dropping bombs. For another joke, Warren made some calcium carbide, which explodes upon contact with water, wrapped it in a slowly water soluble material, uncapped a pipe in his neighbor's swimming pool system, and inserted his package. Later, deep in the heart of the piping, the wrapper dissolved, the calcium carbide blew up, and the neighbor, besides being hysterical with fright, had to have his pool completely replumbed.

During this recitation, Warren seemed as if he were describing something unrelated to himself, like a story he had read about somebody else and was just sharing with the group for their amusement. Healthy anxiety was totally lacking.

In the behind-the-back phase, Bud Bush, somewhat disdainfully, opened with the comment that Warren's story reminded him of a mad scientist yarn in a comic book. The group then settled down to a serious analysis. Their major conclusions were:

1. Warren's "jokes" were not inspired by humor, but, rather, by anger and jealousy, probably of his musically inclined, bright, younger brother whom Warren described as "babied too much."
2. Warren's jokes are vicious and dangerous.
3. Jokes that may hurt somebody are not funny.
4. Warren is play-acting at being a chemist instead of facing up to the hard work that is necessary to become a real one.
5. People should not use their talents to hurt people, as Warren does, but should use them constructively to help make the world a better place.
6. Warren's jokes seemed to be a form of rebellion.
7. Warren did not reveal much of himself to the group, apparently because he does not yet trust the members.
8. Warren seems to be trying to fool himself, masking vicious hostile acts as jokes and making up phony justifications, avoiding recognition of the seriousness of his behavior.
9. Warren would be better off to release his anger through more conventional channels such as playing rough sports.
10. Warren is really angry at his parents and takes it out on innocent strangers, his joke victims.

In the rebuttal phase, Warren tried to defend his position and deny the group's interpretations, but felt the need to continue when the hour closed. He wanted to be subject again next week, but Bud Bush said that he wants a turn. Bud told Warren that he should wait until those who have not been the subject of a meeting get a crack at it before taking a second turn. Warren yielded reluctantly.

SESSION #4 NOTES

Bud Bush described his troubles historically, starting at about age twelve when his mother fell ill and could not work, precipitating desertion by his alcoholic stepfather. Bud took over the role of man of the house, nursing his mother, collecting the aid checks, bringing in a little money from mowing lawns, and, in general, managing the household. He carried out these responsibilities for about two years, enjoying his elevated status, and developing a deep relationship with his mother which in many ways more closely resembled a husband-wife relationship than one between son and mother.

When his mother regained her health and resumed working, Bud found himself both demoted and unsupervised. At this point, he began staying away from home, committing burglaries, assaults, and robberies, bringing home to his mother a lot of money. Among his troubles, Bud was most grieved by his mother's discovery, upon his apprehension, that the money he had been giving her was stolen.

In recent months the stepfather has returned to the home. He is no longer drinking. A remarriage is in the offing.

The behind-the-back phase brought forth the following observations, interpretations and speculations:

1. Bud had a strong desire to demonstrate the loyalty and perseverance that his stepfather lacked.
2. He resented his stepfather's inadequate performance as man of the house, and enjoyed showing him up after he deserted.
3. Bud resented the man of the house privileges his stepfather received without earning them, while he, Bud, earned them after his stepfather's flight, but only received part of them, and then lost those when his mother got well.
4. Bud was elevated prematurely to a position of high responsibility and esteem, lost it when his mother recovered, then tried to regain it by bringing home greater sums of money.
5. He probably really wanted to help his mother, but stealing money for her was a pretty poor way to do it.
6. At his age, just entering his teens, especially in view of the strains brought on by the dissolution of the family and his being forced to assume too much responsibility, Bud desperately needed parental attention and supervision when his mother returned to work, and there was none. Thus, unhappy about his loss of status, and unsupervised, Bud struck out blindly into the world to relieve his feelings in any way that he could.
7. Bud is a nice guy, likeable, and easy to get along with.

8. These comments involve a lot of guessing because, although Bud told his story honestly and sincerely, it did not reveal a very clear picture of him as a person, or what his feelings were about what happened.
9. Bud and his mother will have to be extremely careful in their relationship with the stepfather if the remarriage takes place according to plan. The situation is very touchy, and a cynical comment from either Bud or his mother about the stepfather's desertion, even in a momentary outburst of anger, could upset the family applecart, perhaps driving the stepfather to seek refuge again in the bottle.
10. Bud should weigh his impulses very carefully before acting them out because his hurt feelings about being demoted, and resentment of his stepfather, could cause Bud to do something rash, and in a very short time get himself into trouble again.

Bud readdressed the group, clarified some points and expressed an attitude of forgiveness and friendship for his stepfather. The underlying anger interpreted by the group, however, emerged briefly when Bud blurted, "But if he starts drinking again, I'll kill him."

Glen Grant noted a similarity between Bud's problem and his own rivalry with his stepfather. The group discussed masculine rivalry and posed the question as to why men feel compelled to compete in this way, always trying to prove themselves better than others. I reflected, "It doesn't make much sense to you to get bent out of shape with jealousy. So, some guy is more attractive to a particular woman than you are. So what? Tastes vary. Who can expect to be number one at everything all the time?"

Warren Krist volunteered to be subject again next time.

SESSION #5 NOTES

Glen Grant announced that he wanted to withdraw from the group. I said that he could do that if he wanted to, but I would appreciate hearing his reasons. He said that he did not want to discuss it in the group. I said, "Okay. Do you want to stay for this meeting or leave now?" He said, "I have to stay for this meeting, don't I?'' I said, ''No. This group is purely voluntary. You can quit any time you want to.'' Glen sat down.

The other group members immediately asked Glen why he wanted to quit. He explained that a staff member on his cottage told him that he failed his last classification and was not referred to parole only because he was in my group. I said, ''That is not true, Glen. I did tell the staffing group that you seem to be enjoying, and getting something out of our meetings, but I did not recommend that you be held over just to attend them. The group laughingly pointed out to Glen that he had failed six classifications before he ever joined the group. ''So now, suddenly it's the group's fault?''

Glen continued to express suspicions that I had sold him out. I reflected his feelings and assured him that he is free to stay in the group or leave it, whichever he feels is best for him. I asked if he would like me to dig out my copy of the notes (written by a living-unit staff member) of his classification and read them aloud so we could hear exactly what was said about him. Though reluctant to have his staffing notes read in front of the group, the others urged him on, and he acquiesced.

The notes, of course, contained nothing to support Glen's suspicions that I had prevented his referral to parole in order to keep him in my group. Rather, they described Glen's improving schoolwork, social adjustment and emotional stability. They also stated that he has not yet resolved his problem of boasting and constantly trying to ''prove'' what a big man he is.

By this time it was too late to carry out the behind-the-back process. We filled out the hour with group-centered discussion, still focused on Glen. The other members agreed that Glen's tendency not to trust, or believe in, people probably is a product of past hurts from people he trusted. Glen said that he will decide before next week whether to continue in the group or quit.

Warren Krist will be our subject next time.

SESSION #6 NOTES

Glen decided to continue, and received a warm welcome from the others.

Warren, in his second turn as subject, again blandly recited some of his antisocial adventures. A boastful air in regard to his outsmarting people permeated his narrative, which this time was devoted more to stealing than to "pranks." Evident to me in the incidents he described was the lack of parental strength in setting and enforcing limits on his behavior. Time and again, Warren described his parents' reactions to his thefts, deceptions and disobedience as weak, futile nagging which served only as an irritant.

In the behind-the-back phase, the group went to work on Warren in earnest. They made the following points:

1. Warren deludes himself by playing down the seriousness of his actions. He is fooling himself, but not the rest of the world.
2. He seems to detach himself from the acts he committed, reciting them as entertaining literature not related to him as a person.
3. No practical reason for his stealing is apparent, since his parents gave him anything his heart desired.
4. Perhaps his thieving was just a game aimed at proving he could outsmart someone.
5. He was *not* very smart as a thief, even if this were a desirable trait, since his "cleverness" in getting acquainted and friendly with his victims just before the thefts made him the immediate number one suspect.
6. Warren is not at all smart in wasting his high intelligence childishly irritating people when he could be using it to prepare for really contributing something to the world and helping people.
7. His parents gave him too much and made no real demands on him, so he never learned to assume any responsibility.
8. Warren takes advantage of his parents, easily evading their attempts to control him. Thus, he has no respect for them, and feels no obligation to be honest with them. He relates to them only in terms of getting what he can from them.
9. During his childhood (according to Bud Bush), Warren needed a size ten shoe planted firmly on his butt the first, and every, time he attempted to lie, steal, or show disrespect for his parents.

10. Warren is trying to gain recognition both through his antisocial acts and by his bragging about them. The recognition he gets, though, isn't worth much. The group members do not like him any more for these activities.
11. He is trying to use his bizarre adventures to gain prestige in the group, but the other members tend to gather from Warren's stories that he is "nuts."
12. Warren may have won a few battles toward being a "big wheel" with his "clever" acts, but he is losing the war, since he is locked up and everyone sees him as "a very *little* wheel and a punk."
13. It is questionable whether Warren is really trying to help himself in this group. He seems to be trying just to entertain, and to justify his behavior. Consequently, he is not making any progress toward improving his ability to adjust in the outside community, and will probably get locked up again very soon.

Warren, pale and visibly upset, attempted to defend himself and his parents after I repeated the group's comments to him. He ended his rebuttal with the revelation that his father actually did "beat" him once. The group roared with laughter. Bud Bush exclaimed, "Once! Man, you should have had your ass kicked every time you pulled one of those. You better straighten up before it is too late. You are going to run into a man one of these days who won't go for it. He will sit there and listen while you talk your way out of it, and then say, 'Yes. Very clever. Twenty years.'"

Warren stayed after the meeting to tell me that he thinks he needs to intensify his treatment. He requested transfer into the Escalon program.

The group, very loud and friendly, put pressure on quiet Floyd Walters to be next week's "victim." Blushing, he agreed.

SESSION #7 NOTES

As the group arrived, Floyd Walters approached me with a panicky facial expression, murmuring that he would like to talk to me alone. I told him that would not be fair to the others, since the group meeting was scheduled and the members were already here. I offered to talk with him alone after the meeting. He said that he did not want to tell the group about his problems. I said that he didn't have to be subject if he felt so strongly about it, and that we could just have a regular open discussion. He said that he didn't want to say anything at all. I assured him that he is not required to talk at all if he doesn't feel like it.

As soon as Floyd sat down, Bud Bush asked immediately why he didn't want to talk. The rest of the group added pressure to the question. Floyd began turning red, and finally burst out, "My face! That's why." Bud told him there was nothing wrong with his face, to which Floyd replied, "Yes there is." He said no more, but sat, crimson-faced, obviously in great emotional distress. I reflected his unspoken feeling, "Something is hurting you terribly." Floyd burst into tears but still could not speak. The group, extremely sensitive to Floyd's misery, volunteered to go outside so he could talk to me alone.

Floyd tearfully told me that his girlfriend's parents responded to his request to correspond with her by saying that the girl is in the hospital with some undefined illness. He said that he did not know whether she is really sick, or if this is the parents' way of rejecting him as a suitable friend for their daughter. He said that he didn't care too much, if only he knew the truth. Then he said he could ask his mother to investigate, and dropped the subject.

Gaining control of his tears, Floyd asked if he could drop from the group. He explained that he cannot bear to talk about his face and the way people, especially his father, hurt his feelings about it. I said that he can drop out if that is what he really wants, but that I think it would be a big mistake to run away from the group and continue suffering alone. I said, "Floyd, it is awfully hard to talk about some things, but even so, if you can force yourself to get some of it off your chest, it might make you feel a lot better." He agreed to give it a try.

The group returned. I explained that Floyd found it very difficult to talk about himself, but was going to try. The group members reassured Floyd, telling him that they understand how he feels, and that they sincerely want to help him.

Floyd began falteringly. I assisted by reflecting his expressed feelings. He picked up a head of steam, and poured out his misery.

He described his lifetime of rejection and cruel treatment at the hands of his father. He has been beaten unconscious, insulted, criticized constantly, and treated in general as if he were a loathsome animal. He cried again as he talked about his acne. He told the group of his embarrassment, self-loathing, and inability to go out where people might see him. He described the cruelty of peers who call him "syph face," and of his father who constantly hounded him about it. He explained that he has made his parole classification, but is going to ask the Board for a holdover because he cannot bear to see his father until his face is well.

In the behind-the-back phase, the group made the following points:

1. Floyd's dad seems to be "a nut." If he were out of the way, most of Floyd's problems would be solved.
2. The group would like to beat the hell out of Floyd's dad.
3. If Floyd's acne *could* be cleared up medically, it would not solve his problem with his dad, but it would make Floyd a lot more comfortable with himself and others.
4. Floyd's face looks a lot worse to him than it does to them.
5. His father is either "mentally ill" or "just doesn't give a damn."
6. Floyd holds back his pain until it reaches a bursting point. He ought to tell people off the minute they say something to hurt him.
7. The letter from his girlfriend's parents simply served as a trigger for all of the painful feelings Floyd has kept bottled up within himself.
8. Being treated as a worthless person by his father has made Floyd doubt his own worth, and wonder why he is so horrible. He has seized upon the acne as a possible explanation for his "worthlessness," and has in this way become overly sensitive about it.
9. His father has used Floyd as an object of ridicule in order to make himself feel more important and worthwhile. He tries to elevate his own self-esteem by tearing down Floyd's.
10. Floyd's father does not love him, or he would try to get medi-

cal help for the acne, instead of using it as a tool for self-glorification.
11. Floyd ought to consider foster home placement.
12. His mother should have thrown the father out for abusing Floyd, but she probably loves her husband, or is afraid of him, or can't face the issue of having to choose between husband and son.
13. Perhaps I could investigate state resources for possible medical treatment of Floyd's acne.
14. If Floyd had a halfway decent home situation he could get along well "on the outs" because ". . . he is a nice guy, uses his head, and has good sense."
15. Floyd is too modest and quiet, so that people don't get a chance to find out what a really nice guy he is.

Floyd, in his reply, verified the accuracy and wisdom of a number of the group's observations. He explained, however, that he has thought about foster home placement, but can't bear to leave his mother and sisters, whom he loves. One possible exception might be placement with his former employer who lives only a few blocks away, if he would have him.

He said that he would not like to see his father killed, but ". . . only beaten half to death." He was still discharging anger toward his father when the hour closed. He stayed, continuing the tirade for half an hour after the others left, as I reflected his feelings. When I had to close the office, I asked if he would like to return in the morning and continue. He said that he would.*

Mickey Switt volunteered for next week.

SESSION #8 NOTES

Mickey Switt took his first turn as "victim," and narrated his past offenses, ranging from kindergarten mischief to the event for which he was committed, burglary turned into armed robbery when his victim unexpectedly returned home. He employed his usual "cool stud" style of delivery, mixing incongruously the gestures,

---

* And he did for another hour.

terminology and phony "Dead End Kids" accent with the face, voice and occasional inflections of a small boy playing cops and robbers.

Mickey attempted to take personal blame for all of his misfortunes, in what seemed to be a grandstand play for the admiration of the group. He glorified his parents, especially his father, as the best and most beloved in the world. (I detected a note of bitterness in the description of his father's unbelievable brilliance and competence.)

In the behind-the-back phase, Mickey listened to the group slice through his role-playing act as if it were warm butter:

1. Mickey is similar to Warren Krist in that they both try to con people, and pull the wool over their eyes. Neither of them are anywhere near as good at it as they think they are.
2. Mickey's story was hard to decipher. His actions didn't make much sense.
3. His parents actually must love him quite a bit.
4. Mickey seems to have been overprotected, also like Warren, and attempts to gain some independence through his sneaky antisocial acts.
5. He could do just about anything he wanted to without worrying much about consequences, since his parents would try to protect him.
6. He seems to have grown up a little in the institutional setting. He showed some maturity when he took it like a man, instead of "throwing a fit" when institution officials set a limit on the number of visits and gifts he could receive from his parents, who were flooding him with both.
7. Mickey is a nice guy, very likeable.
8. If he goes to school with serious intentions, stays away from alcohol, and continues to grow up in his attitudes, Mickey will make it alright "on the outs."
9. His home situation is one in which Mickey can live quite comfortably if he makes the effort and quits taking advantage of his parents.
10. His past antisocial acts appear to be some form of ". . . trying to show someone up or get attention." (At this point I asked the group if they could think of anybody that Mickey

might be trying to "show up." They said that they could think of nobody, since Mickey is an only child. I asked, "How about his father? Mickey described him being near-perfect in all areas. Maybe he gets tired of having his father outshine him all the time." This didn't seem to mean much to the group, but Mickey responded with an exaggerated cough.)

11. Mickey tries to act like he is "real cool." The acting is apparent. Everyone can tell that he is trying to make himself feel big by playing a role, and this causes people to lose respect for him.

12. His talking "big" is not as bad as the way some guys try to play "cool stud" by pushing people around.

13. Mickey's stories about himself are "built up" (exaggerated) to make him look bigger than he is.

14. If true, his story about deciding to surrender to police without trying to shoot it out showed good judgment.

15. Mickey is taking an unusually long time to "make the program" and earn parole because his defying authority and ignoring rules are lifelong habits.

16. When Mickey does get out, armed with the more mature attitudes he seems to be developing, he will probably be successful.

In the rebuttal period, Mickey said that the group analyzed him pretty accurately. He was especially impressed with my comments about his father always showing him up. He went on to express considerable anger about it, and told the group how much he hates it when his father unfavorably compares Mickey's behavior with ". . . what he did when he was a boy."

Mickey verified that his outlook is becoming more mature. He said that he realizes he must settle down, finish school and achieve something real.

He said that he has more to say about himself, and volunteered to be subject again next week.

SESSION #9 NOTES

Mickey Switt elaborated on his relationship with his father. He described a number of examples of perfectionistic, demanding behavior, but concluded that he doesn't blame his father because his intentions were good — to try to make Mickey a better person. Also, going all out for perfection is his father's approach to everything he does. Mickey pointed out that his father's critical, demanding approach is not aimed at him alone, but also at his mother. He said that his father always flooded his mother with unsolicited instructions at the bowling alley when all she wanted was to bowl for fun and enjoy being with friends.

Mickey was much less dramatic and "cool" in his presentation this week.

The group's behind-the-back observations were the following:

1. Being pushed hard toward high standards is an advantage in some ways. Such a program can produce achievement.
2. There are limits upon the extent to which such demands can be imposed without producing feelings of failure, resentment and rebellion. Mickey has had too many demands made by his father.
3. Mickey gave up trying to meet his father's impossible standards of drive and accomplishment and rebelled by taking a shiftless, lackadaisical attitude toward everything. This has produced delinquent behavior, and very little achievement.
4. He drifted into his negative behavior pattern gradually, starting very young, not realizing where it was leading, or why it was happening, until he suddenly discovered himself in deep and dangerous waters.
5. If Mickey were seeking perfection as a criminal in order to match his father's brilliance in other areas, he didn't succeed, since here he is, locked up.
6. His father's approach to life is not a very good one, in that preoccupation with accomplishment prevents him from enjoying a lot of things, and is the kind of outlook that can cause ulcers.
7. A better balanced approach would be to develop a few talents

as much as possible, and just lean back and enjoy the other areas of life without trying to achieve perfection in them.

8. Mickey's father's quest for absolute perfection in even one area is an impossible one. Excellence, yes. Perfection, no.

9. Accomplishment is a source of satisfaction, but total striving for it may leave no time for the many other satisfactions in life.

10. Total negative refusal to work for accomplishment is just as bad an approach to life as total striving for it. Mickey needs to pick out some goals to work toward, but save some time to kick back and have fun.

11. Drifting into a negative pattern like Mickey's is a lot easier than getting out of it.

12. Mickey is showing more mature thinking than he used to, as evidenced in his ability to accept without anger his father's unrealistic demands upon him, recognizing them as well-intentioned, if misguided.

13. He seems to be on the right track in discussing his feelings freely with his father (which he reported he was able to do for the first time on their last visit). The way to break the old pattern is for each of them to become aware of the other's viewpoints and needs.

Mickey said that he had nothing to say in the rebuttal period. The group used the remaining time to rap about drugs and hypnosis.

Glen Grant volunteered for next week.

CONCLUSION

This group continued for a total of thirty-two meetings, adding two new members along the way to replace those who were paroled (Mickey and Floyd). All of the members had a great many misconceptions corrected about themselves and their ideas about how others perceived their behaviors.

The astuteness of teenagers at evaluating and proposing workable solutions to the problems of their troubled peers has never ceased to amaze me. Here is a tremendous treatment resource, almost never tapped. Instead, many professional therapists, basking in their academic self-exaltation, try to do it all by themselves, spewing profound interpretations which, generally, the teenagers listen to politely, then "throw for a dead shine."

To most teenagers, what their own peers honestly think about them and say about them behind their backs is about a hundred times more important than the opinions of some square, ivy-covered therapist, and another hundred times more effective at inspiring emotional and social growth.

The behind-the-back format can be valuable in many settings other than group therapy with delinquent youths. For instance, it is a remarkable device for increasing staff cohesiveness, mutual understanding, and on-the-job cooperation when used as a training technique. You see, even nominally well adjusted adults can often profit from letting others know how they really see themselves, and finding out how others honest-to-God see them.

NOTE

1. Not being a physicist, I cannot vouch for the technical accuracy of Warren's cyclatron formula. I was not inclined to doubt him, however, in the light of his proven successes with the flamethrower and electric toilet.

Chapter XIX

Community Counseling

Recall from Chapter III that the self-images of youths, especially institutionalized delinquents, are often incomplete. Lacking the variety of interpersonal experiences which would have taught them who they are in a wide range of social contexts, they live in very limited worlds. Some know who they are only as individuals ("Me, myself and I."). Others have practically no sense of individuality ("a boy; a human being; something living"), and see themselves as blurry ill-defined somethings drifting along in a confusing world of other vague shadows. Some can identify themselves only as members of a family. Others never had much of a family and have no sense of existence in the context of a small, intimate, sharing group. Some had no adequate relationship with nurturing parents and have no concept of participating in an intimate one-to-one relationship. Others can experience themselves as individuals, as members of a family type group, but not as members of a larger meaningful community, or of an occupational group.

It was postulated that a wholesome group living program for such people must include structured opportunities for them to relate to others, and thereby learn who they are at the levels of intimacy which are lacking in their individual self-concepts. A number of traditional institutional programs can contribute to this cause. Classroom instruction and trade training, for instance, can develop a sense of identity as a scholar or as a member of an occupational group in those who are deficient in those areas. The thrust of this book, however, has been the description and illustration of techniques designed *specifically* to stimulate emotional and social growth, and to extend self-concepts into levels of intimacy in which they have never before dwelt.

We have covered thus far the ingredients of a growth-producing, as opposed to stifling, atmosphere in the overall living environment (*milieu* therapy). We have discussed the rationale and techniques for, and illustrated, several varieties of effective individual, or one-to-one therapy. We have done the same for systems designed to provide growth-stimulating experiences in the context of a small, intimate, sharing group.

The subject of this chapter, community counseling, adds the final dimension to what must be provided as a minimum by any institution or group living program wishing to call itself a treatment facility.[1] If half of these services are provided, we have a semi-treatment facility. If none of them are provided, we have a holding pen for disturbed people, which would be more suitable for cattle.

Community counseling consists of *regular* meetings of all staff and residents of a specific living unit. In a small facility this might be the whole institution. A large institution might contain a dozen living units of a hundred residents each. That large institution should have twelve community counseling programs.

Many of the elements of small group counseling are applicable to the community meeting; but the two differ in a number of ways. They are similar in that they are both democratically oriented, subject matter being determined by the group itself. Community meetings differ from small group in size (a hundred or more members sometimes); frequency (daily meetings if possible); content (more concrete problems of daily community living and less intimate personal material); and membership (a mixture of all staff and residents of the community).

In addition to providing personal growth opportunity for members (staff as well as residents), community meetings as a management tool provide staff with a side benefit which in itself justifies the program. The introduction of community meetings in every instance has produced a reduction of antisocial and violent behavior among the residents.

A yearlong formal research conducted by Stuart Adams for the California Youth Authority at the Paso Robles School clearly verified the preceding statement. The residents of four living units (fifty each) were measured on a number of variables during the institutional phase of the research, after which they were followed up on parole for several years. One living unit provided only small group (group-centered) counseling once per week for all residents. A second unit featured community meetings only (two per week). A third provided both small group and community counseling. The fourth, the control unit, provided neither. The residents of the two units with community counseling programs received significantly fewer discipline reports, spent significantly less lock-up time in the discipline unit, and had a significantly lower percentage of incidents involving violence than did the residents of the other two units. Results for the small-group-only unit were superior on all of these variables to those of the no-group-counseling-at-all unit.[2]

Staff on the units which employed it reported enthusiastically that community counseling was an extremely valuable part of the residents' group living experience, as well as a boon to morale and the smoothness of cottage management. At the close of the formal research period, the superintendent instructed me to start immediately to develop community counseling programs on the six living units which had none. (Escalon-Nipomo had the first, but was not included in the research due to the selected, emotionally disturbed population and the number of other specialized treatment techniques already being employed there.)

The role of the leader is crucial to the success of community meetings. Some staff are just not emotionally or intellectually equipped to handle it, even after training. That is why I personally selected the group leader and an alternate from the staff of each unit and trained them intensively, including demonstrating by leading their meetings for a month. That is also why the rest of this chapter will be devoted largely to the leader's outlook and techniques.

Creating the proper atmosphere for large group community counseling is often difficult in the traditional military-like setting of an institution. The role which the community meeting leader must assume is almost the exact opposite of that of the military officer, which conveys, "I am the boss. I have the authority. You are of little significance except to follow my orders." The community meeting leader's role communicates, "This is *our* community. We each have an individual place in our community, but we interrelate and help each other to solve our mutual problems. We cooperate to make our community a better place to live."

The distinctions between these two roles, while essential to the success of a growth-inducing group program, are not always easy to grasp. Sometimes staff, in attempting to adopt this "sharing" attitude, swing too far on the pendulum and abdicate their authority. They assume that to be a democratic leader one must give up being himself, and permit the residents to behave in any way they choose. To be sure, this is just as far from the proper attitude for a community group leader as is, "I am the boss. Obey me, or else!"

At no time should any of the staff members in a community meeting give up any of their authority. They just refrain from flaunting it. In fact, they *must* retain their authority in order for the meetings to provide one of their major benefits. Many youths have a stereotyped concept of authority as being punitive, rigid, demanding, and aloof or rejecting. Staff members, through *retaining* their authority in a community meeting and employing it *in a warm, accepting, understanding and fair way*, actually force these youths to recognize the inaccuracy of their views of authority, and correct them.

The leader, in particular, does not attack or criticize a resident for expressing antisocial, distorted or angry feelings. Neither does he ignore this kind of behavior. Rather, he focuses the attention of the group upon it, enlisting their aid in bringing about improved understanding and solutions to the problem behaviors.

Physically, a room big enough to seat the whole community in a circular arrangement is required. All participants must be able to see each others' faces. In institutions, living unit dayrooms are usually used.

As with group-centered small group counseling, the community will eventually learn more about the operation and purpose of the large meetings from the leader's actions than from any formal introductory speech. However, due to the size of the community meeting, an introductory statement of purpose and ground rules is advisable. The leader may wish to begin the first meeting with a statement similar to the following:

> Living and working together in a large group as we do produces problems. That is natural. It is not easy to rub elbows with so many people twenty-four hours a day and get along with them always. Frictions are bound to arise.

Additionally, each of us has problems which we brought into this situation with us—personal problems, problems in getting along with others, with teachers, with the police, with the family at home. These kinds of problems, and those that arise from group living, always make somebody unhappy and angry.

There are two general approaches to trying to solve such problems. When a person is angry or unhappy he may break something or attack somebody, which is likely to bring him even more trouble. The alternative is for him to talk about his problem, try to identify and let others know what is bothering him, and work with them to find a solution to the problem which will not cause him more trouble.

In our living unit we are going to have regular meetings, like this one, of the whole community. The purpose is to give us a way and a place to work out those problems sensibly, and to make life more pleasant for everybody in the program.

In these meetings, any member of this group may talk about any problem he chooses. Although everyone will be expected to attend, no one is required to participate in the discussion. Anyone who just wants to listen courteously may do so, but anyone who feels like putting his two cents worth into the discussions will be welcome. Our one iron-clad rule is that the group is meeting so that we may help, not hurt each other. Now, what have you got on your minds?

In attempting to define the role of the leader, let me reemphasize that he is an authority figure with full authority who employs it in a kindly, fair and understanding way. He is not a weak, passive, namby-pamby who ignores unpleasant, hostile, or threatening emotional behavior within the group. Neither is he a rigid dictator who forbids the expression of "hot" or "loaded" material. Both the lax, passive leader, and the rigid dictator are afraid to face and deal with the unpleasant feelings expressed by the group members.

What *is* required of the community counseling leader is enough personal inner security to permit him to listen calmly and objectively to the expression of angry, threatening feelings, perhaps inquire further into their meaning, to help the group recognize and understand the problems being expressed, and to guide (not direct) them in developing solutions.

The term "permissiveness" frequently causes confusion (and arguments). People sometimes equate it with laxity, with passivity, and the complete absence of discipline. To professionals in group dynamics, that is not at all what the term means. Rather, a "permissive atmosphere" in a group means that the members feel free to express their feelings verbally, not to *do* anything they choose. A permissive leader permits his group members to express feelings, *any feelings*, verbally. This does not imply that he condones or permits their expression in overt behavior.

Many situations develop in community counseling which require quick, skillful, spontaneous solutions by the group leader. Let us take a random look at some such situations. Hopefully, discussion of a few samples will help new group leaders to formulate a general frame of reference, a kind of basic position, or stance, from which to approach the management challenges which will unpredictably pop up from time to time in their own meetings.

HANDLING FRIVOLOUS
ADMINISTRATIVE QUESTIONS

One common problem is what to do about frivolous administrative questions brought up in the community counseling session. The purpose of the meeting is the discussion and solution of personal, emotional and social problems in the context of the group living community. How does the leader deal with questions such as, "Why doesn't the institution let us have visitors any time of the day?" or "Why can't we have breakfast served in bed?"

A leader can quickly train his group not to bring up such unproductive subject matter by ignoring the questions (remaining silent, or asking the group if they have anything they would like to discuss). This is probably the best approach.

Frequent occurrence of administrative complaints in the community meetings often point up a need for a student government system in the community. If the residents elect a council of representatives who can have a voice in the administration of their own program, they will not need to try to use community counseling for this purpose. (Further, such a system sets up another area of interpersonal experience which residents can use to add a new dimension to their self-concepts.)

DEALING WITH THE SELF-CENTERED POWER-STRIVER

Another common, and very thorny problem encountered in conducting meetings of this size is the attention-seeking, hostile, egocentric power-striver who attempts to take control of the group for his own purposes. (Remember Lenny Coyle in the chapter illustrating small group-centered counseling?) In community counseling, such a character inevitably appears and makes his play to use the meeting as his own private showcase, or destroy it. The leader cannot ignore this, or soon he will have no meeting to lead. Neither can he throttle the culprit and have him hauled off to lock-up, or he will be violating his own freedom of speech ground rules.

What can the leader do? He can do what the group leader is supposed to do. He can deal with these manipulations in the same way he responds to any other feelings or thoughts expressed by a group member. He can meet them head on gently and without counter-hostility. He can ask what the attention-seeker's statement means, how the rest of the group feels about the situation, whether it poses a threat to the group, whether the initial ground rule of "helping, not hurting each other" is being observed, and what the individual and the rest of the group feel might be done to solve it if it is a problem.

To illustrate, the leader might say to a member who has been monopolizing the meeting time to express irrelevancies, sarcasm, or whatever suits his selfish interests, and intimidating others who tried to speak, "It appears that you don't want the others in the group to speak." Frequently, a simple statement of fact such as this will stop the disruptive behavior. At other times the "offender" may push the issue further. If so the leader, still calmly and courteously, must make his confrontation a little stronger, perhaps asking, "Do you feel that the other members should not be allowed to express their opinions, and only you should?" Or he could ask,

"Might you be trying to use the group to entertain yourself, or put yourself in the limelight?"

By this time, usually, one or more other members of the group are trying eagerly to enter the discussion on the side of fair play. The majority want the group to be used for its original purpose, everybody helping one another, not for the one individual to take it over for his own purposes. These peers can, and do, confront the manipulator with much more point-blank disapproval than the leader may express in his role. At the right moment, the leader may call in these reinforcements by saying, "Joe, you have been trying to say something about this. What have you got on your mind?" Joe, and probably a couple of other members, will set the manipulator straight in no uncertain terms.

In the extremely rare instances when the takover artist has not been subdued at this point, the leader can call in the cavalry. The strongest force in the meeting is pressure from the entire community. The leader may address the entire assembly (staff included), "How do the rest of you feel about this? Although the main purpose of this meeting is for all of us to express our feelings and help each other find solutions to problems, Sam Jones here seems to be of the opinion that he alone should decide what we can talk about and who is allowed to speak. We can run the meetings either way, so that *everyone* has a voice in our community, or the way Sam wants it — he decides who can express their opinions and who can't. It's our community, and these are our meetings. We can run them however we please. How do you want it to be?" I have never seen a wise guy power-striver continue his campaign after the weight of the total community fell on him.

SUBGROUP ABUSE OF THE MEETING

Sometimes the power-seeking show-off picks up supporters who help him in his attempt to pervert the meeting's purpose. When this happens, the leader deals with it in the same basic way, simply pointing out and interpreting what is happening. He might comment, "It appears that several of you want to use our meeting to make fun of and put down others in the group. I wonder if this might not be a violation of our agreement that the purpose of these meetings is to help, not hurt, each other. What do the rest of you think?"

Again, the role of the leader is that of the fair, benevolent, but very *authoritative* (as opposed to "authoritarian" or "autocratic") authority figure. He does not demand; he does not threaten; he does not ignore. He remains sensitive to what is going on and helps the group to understand what is happening. He does not evade "loaded" issues. He does not criticize members of the group for the opinions they express, or even for trying to distort the purpose of the meetings. He faces issues squarely, but objectively, and without malevolence. He involves the whole community in the solutions to their own problems.

VERBAL ATTACKS ON FELLOW STAFF WHO ARE NOT PRESENT

Leaders often experience conflict when wards express hostile or insulting opinions about other staff who are not present to defend themselves. Traditionally, staff are expected to defend staff, no matter what. In community counseling the leader may not do this. His noncritical role as leader does not permit him to take sides and play defense attorney for his colleagues. His primary responsibility is to encourage the members of his group to express their feelings, as angry, distorted, bizarre, inappropriate or illogical as they may seem. He may reflect back the expressed feelings, encouraging the member to move forward in his own quest for self-understanding.[3] He may turn to the group for a broader sampling of opinion, saying, "Tom here feels that school teacher Doe is always unfair and deliberately picks on him — that when he gets a low grade it is not because of what he did, but because Mr. Doe doesn't like him. How do the rest of you feel about this? Do you think that the low grades are based entirely on personal dislike for Tom, or might there be other factors involved?"

By remaining neutral, rather than siding with Tom or defending teacher Doe, the leader puts himself in a position to lead his group members to some valuable improvements in their own attitudes and self-concepts. Objective, noncritical discussion of one group member's negative feelings and attitudes often leads other group members to recognize and correct their own prejudiced, stereotyped attitudes, and tendencies to blame everyone in the world but themselves for their troubles. It is much easier for a community member to recognize a faulty attitude in a peer and then ask himself, "Am I like that too?" than it is to accept a direct, critical statement from staff that he *is* like that.

PROFANITY/OBSCENITY

The group leader, knowing that the agency for whom he works officially disapproves of the use of profanity and/or obscenity*, finds himself in a quandary when the members of his group use it. Having guaranteed the community freedom of expression, he is now faced with the question, "Shall I renege on this guarantee or shall I permit them to use this language even though my employer officially disapproves of it?" The basic answer to this question is that the agency which employs the group leader approves of community counseling (or he wouldn't be leading it), and community counseling, by definition, *requires* freedom of expression. Practically speaking, then, the agency need not abandon its official disapproval of foul language, but it must waive its customary direct and autocratic (and ineffective) prohibition of such language in order to permit free communication in the meetings. If the agency will not take this position, the leader must either lead less-than-adequate, crippled, community counseling, or find work elsewhere.

If genuine and important feelings are expressed, clothed in profane words, the leader is remiss if he changes the focus from the feelings to the profanity. This is shortsighted, pedantic preaching, not counseling.

There are times, however, when the salty language is of more importance to the individual than the ideas he pretends to be expressing. The use of profanity may become an end in itself. At such times it is the responsibility of the leader to point out this possibility, and to inquire of the individual and the group as to what it might mean. Perhaps it is aimed at some members (or visitors) whom he is

---

*Though they've never been able to stop it.

trying to impress. It may symbolize contempt, sexual exhibitionism, or any number of other attitudes. The leader may legitimately ask the group to explore such areas.

Many times overuse of foul language symbolizes angry feelings toward authority in general, or the group leader in particular. One common situation which can produce this kind of hostility is for staff to bring visitors to the meeting without first having asked the group's permission, or at least explaining in advance who the visitors are and why they are visiting. When unannounced visitors are brought in members tend to feel that *their* meeting is being violated by strangers. Some of them express a feeling that they are being put on display by the leader, and that he is more interested in showing off his community meetings than in actually helping them. They often curse up a storm.

Once again, the leader does not attack group members for using profanity/obscenity, nor does he ignore it if it is of such proportions that it overshadows the subject matter under discussion. The leader should be objective and personally secure enough to face up to such language in a calm, realistic way, not permitting it to cloud more important issues, nor ignoring it when the language itself takes on symptomatic importance.

MISCELLANEOUS

Other common problem situations that arise in community counseling include threats of violence; passive defiance of the ground rules (e.g., a member reading a magazine, or a small subgroup talking privately and ignoring what is going on in the main group); and verbal insults directed at the leader. The leader, hopefully, will handle each of these annoying incidents in a calm, mature, inquiring way. Never relinquishing his authority, he must employ it kindly, but firmly, to resolve such crises.

To the member reading a magazine, he may say at an appropriate opportunity, "You seem to be avoiding the discussion today. Why?" or, if the resistance continues, "You do not have to talk if you don't want to, but remember our ground rule that everybody is expected to be courteous and pay attention to those who do have something to say."

To a member who threatens to punch another one, the leader calmly comments, "Our rule is that we may say anything we want in this meeting, but we do not hit people." (Should a member actually strike in violence, the leader must ask present staff to remove the offender immediately.)

To say that the leader should never become angry in a meeting is unrealistic. However, it is quite realistic, and desirable for him to be able to express such emotions calmly and rationally. Such a demonstration of self-control is essentially valuable to members who have hostility-control problems of their own, and look to the leader as a role model. It is much more useful for the leader to admit his anger and demonstrate that he can control it than to pretend he is a superhuman who never has negative emotions. If directly insulted by a member, the leader can say, "That hurts my feelings, John, and it really makes me angry. I don't believe it is justified. Can you tell me why you think it is?"

Very few actual persons, if any, are identical to the ideal group leader described in this chapter. Some individuals are more comfortable with a more passive, laissez-faire approach, while others feel a strong need to display their authority in more concrete ways. Such personality differences do not prohibit useful results in community counseling. Leaning too far in either direction, however, reduces effectiveness.

One cannot become an effective community counseling leader by reading alone. This chapter can be of introductory value only. Growth as a group leader can take place only through experiencing (and sweating) the group process, pondering and discussing these experiences, evaluating and reevaluating one's own feelings and responses to the myriad situations and problems that emerge in the meetings. Brief "critique" meetings of staff following the community sessions are valuable.

Administrators of group living programs who wish to enhance the value of their programs, and reduce frictions, would do well to hire a professional to come in, establish a demonstration group, and use it to train key staff in the leadership role. In this way, in a short time the facility can develop its own internal resources and provide its own expertise.

In any personality counseling, individual, small group, or community, only a small proportion of the time is actually devoted to so-called "important" subject matter. The most important growth-producing factor is not what is said, but the atmosphere in which it is said. This atmosphere is determined by the warmth, sensitivity, understanding and social courage of the counselor. All people have an infinite capacity to continue growing in these areas.

NOTES

1. Critics sometimes say, "Institutional treatment is a waste of time. It doesn't work." The only time it doesn't work, which is often, is when it hasn't been tried, or has been tried incompetently.

2. This pattern was paralleled in the parole follow-up. Parolees from the community meeting units had lower recidivism rates.

3. Remember that negative feelings must be expressed, recognized by the listener, and cleared out of the way before the positive and rational attitudes on the issue can emerge. One cannot see positives when he is choked with anger.

Chapter XX

Some People I Learned From
(Or, From Whom, If You Prefer)

As I mentioned earlier, I never came up with anything original in my whole life, except original ways to reintegrate the "original" ideas of others.*

Thousands have contributed to my frame of reference. I can't remember them all. Right now, though, there are a few who flash across my mind. Most of their names are well known to folks in the people-helping business, so all I'm going to do is mention a paraphrased concept or two from each that contributed most to my eclectic approach to treatment. If you want to know more about their thinking, their works are in libraries and book stores everywhere:

1. Provide a fertile, growth-encouraging atmosphere by noncritically reflecting feelings, and the client's inner resources will mobilize themselves to find solutions to his own problems. *Carl Rogers*
2. The delinquent is locked up not primarily because his childhood relationships with his parents were conflict-ridden. He is locked up because he committed a crime. That is the place to start in reality therapy. *William Glasser*
3. A symptom is formed when a basic, legitimate human need is blocked from direct expression by a traumatic experience. The therapist may approach his task by digging in the unconscious

---

*Theirs weren't original, either. They just reintegrated somebody else's nonoriginal ideas into original mixtures that got the job done a little better. That's what I've tried to do.

for the trauma (psychoanalysis); by focusing on characterological or strategic defenses against reemergence of the original need in undisguised form (character analysis and neoanalysis); by attacking the symptom itself (behavior modification and hypnotic suggestion); or by focusing upon, and reflecting the painful feelings spawned by the process (client-centered therapy). Another little recognized approach, and probably the quickest and most effective one, is to identify the blocked need and present it for evaluation in a form that allows satisfaction of it in a non-symptomatic, non-traumatic way. If the legitimate need is gratified, the symptom no longer has a purpose, and disappears. (The basis for my "Why Not?" therapy.) As far as I know, the concept was developed by *Vance Boileau.*

4. Nobody has the power to hurt you directly with words. The only one who can hurt you *is you* through what you say to yourself *about* what someone else says to you.
   Albert Ellis

5. Clear thinking techniques can be taught, and through this process, adult intelligence can be increased.
   Albert Upton

6. People can say things and listen to things when out of eye contact that they can't tolerate face-to-face. (A key principle in the behind-the-back group therapy technique.)
   Sigmund Freud and his couch

7. The large group community meeting can help to sanitize the oppressive atmosphere of an institution and provide a forum for socially acceptable solutions to the problems arising from group living.
   Glynn Smith

8. In some cases, hypnoanalytic techniques can be used to cut through defenses and reduce treatment time by months.
   Lewis Wolberg

9. The "therapeutic community," in unscrupulous or ignorant hands, can be perverted into a sham program that is far more detrimental to the residents than no program at all.
   Novelist *Ken Kesey (One Flew Over the Cuckoo's Nest)*

Now, I'm going to close by listing some of the people who *really* taught me the things I needed to know to write this book.

Withdrawn Willie
Heinous Harry
Twister Thompson
Little Hitler Smally
Sow's Ear Lee
Suicidal Jake Best
Buck Douglas, Murder in the Making
J.D. Boothe
Jim Caven
Lenny Coyle
Del Swanson
Pat Muldoon
Bud Bush
Glen Grant
Mickey Switt
Floyd Walters
Warren Krist*

---

*If your swimming pool hasn't blown up lately, or your hedge hasn't been incinerated by a flame thrower, or nobody has been electrocuted on your toilet, you'll probably want to thank me for at least partially accomplishing my mission. Warren is a *real* chemist now.